Understanding Research for Nursing Students

Transforming Nursing Practice series

Transforming Nursing Practice is the first series of books designed to help students meet the requirements of the NMC Standards and Essential Skills Clusters for degree programmes. Each book addresses a core topic, and together they cover the generic knowledge required for all fields of practice. Accessible and challenging, *Transforming Nursing Practice* helps nursing students prepare for the demands of future healthcare delivery.

Core knowledge titles:

Series editor: Professor Shirley Bach, Head of the School of Nursing and Midwifery at the University of Brighton

Acute and Critical Care in Adult Nursing	ISBN 978 0 85725 842 7
Becoming a Registered Nurse: Making the Transition to Practice	ISBN 978 0 85725 931 8
Communication and Interpersonal Skills in Nursing (2nd edn)	ISBN 978 0 85725 449 8
Contexts of Contemporary Nursing (2nd edn)	ISBN 978 1 84445 374 0
Dementia Care in Nursing	ISBN 978 0 85725 873 1
Getting into Nursing	ISBN 978 0 85725 895 3
Health Promotion and Public Health for Nursing Students	ISBN 978 0 85725 437 5
Introduction to Medicines Management in Nursing	ISBN 978 1 84445 845 5
Law and Professional Issues in Nursing (2nd edn)	ISBN 978 1 84445 372 6
Leadership, Management and Team Working in Nursing	ISBN 978 0 85725 453 5
Learning Skills for Nursing Students	ISBN 978 1 84445 376 4
Medicines Management in Adult Nursing	ISBN 978 1 84445 842 4
Medicines Management in Children's Nursing	ISBN 978 1 84445 470 9
Medicines Management in Mental Health Nursing	ISBN 978 0 85725 049 0
Mental Health Law in Nursing	ISBN 978 0 85725 863 2
Nursing Adults with Long Term Conditions	ISBN 978 0 85725 441 2
Nursing and Collaborative Practice (2nd edn)	ISBN 978 1 84445 373 3
Nursing and Mental Health Care	ISBN 978 1 84445 467 9
Passing Calculations Tests for Nursing Students (2nd edn)	ISBN 978 1 4465 642 8
Patient and Carer Participation in Nursing	ISBN 978 0 85725 307 1
Patient Assessment and Care Planning in Nursing	ISBN 978 0 85725 858 8
Psychology and Sociology in Nursing	ISBN 978 0 85725 836 6
Safeguarding Adults in Nursing Practice	ISBN 978 1 44625 638 1
Successful Practice Learning for Nursing Students (2nd edn)	ISBN 978 0 85725 315 6
Using Health Policy in Nursing	ISBN 978 1 44625 646 6
What is Nursing? Exploring Theory and Practice (3rd edn)	ISBN 978 0 85725 975 2

Personal and professional learning skills titles:

Series editors: Dr Mooi Standing, Independent Academic Consultant (UK and International) and Accredited NMC Reviewer and Professor Shirley Bach, Head of the School of Nursing and Midwifery at the University of Brighton

Clinical Judgement and Decision Making in Nursing	ISBN 978 1 84445 468 6
Critical Thinking and Writing for Nursing Students (2nd edn)	ISBN 978 1 44625 644 2
Evidence-based Practice in Nursing (2nd edn)	ISBN 978 1 44627 090 5
Information Skills for Nursing Students	ISBN 978 1 84445 381 8
Reflective Practice in Nursing (2nd edn)	ISBN 978 1 44627 085 1
Succeeding in Essays, Exams and OSCEs for Nursing Students	ISBN 978 0 85725 827 4
Succeeding in Research Project Plans and Literature Reviews for Nursing Students	ISBN 978 0 85725 264 7
Successful Professional Portfolios for Nursing Students	ISBN 978 0 85725 457 3
Understanding Research for Nursing Students (2nd edn)	ISBN 978 1 44626 761 5

You can find more information on each of these titles and our other learning resources at **www.sagepub.co.uk**. Many of these titles are also available in various e-book formats; please visit our website for more information.

Contents

Foreword

The *Transforming Nursing Practice* series includes several titles that focus on personal and professional learning skills, and *Understanding Research for Nursing Students* is a key text in this respect. On a personal level, it offers students opportunities to gain confidence by getting to grips with important aspects of the research process in nursing. On a professional level, it succinctly demonstrates how a wide range of research methods are used to generate knowledge that can be applied to enhance the quality of care that service users receive. It promotes an awareness of uncertainty, what we don't know and what we need to find out in order to provide the best care possible. In this way the book encourages students to adopt a healthy questioning approach to their everyday care of patients. This also goes hand in hand with lifelong learning and their continuing personal and professional development as nurses. The book gives lots of practical examples and illustrations to help readers relate to the topic, and there are numerous activities to engage with, test out ideas and deepen understanding. After reading this book, students should have a good grasp of research that will help them both in their academic work and in contributing to evidence-based practical nursing care.

In the second edition of this popular book Peter Ellis has incorporated changes that take account of new developments, reviews and readers' feedback. Some concepts such as the research process are described in more detail. Many recently published nursing research studies are described. This highlights how nursing research is continually developing and the need for nurses to keep updated in this respect. The variety of studies referred to also helps to broaden the book's appeal as it enables nursing students from all pathways to relate to research to their area of clinical practice. The new chapter on using research gives a useful snapshot into the contribution that research can make to high quality evidence-based care.

Dr Mooi Standing
Series Editor

About the author

Peter Ellis is Senior Lecturer in Nursing and Applied Clinical Studies at Canterbury Christ Church University, where he is also Programme Director for Health and Social Care Continuing Professional Development: Interprofessional Practice and Departmental Lead for Partnership and Internationalisation. Peter teaches research, kidney care and leadership and management at all levels of study. Peter has a first degree in Nursing and higher degrees in Health Care Ethics and Medical Epidemiology. Peter has been publishing in professional journals and textbooks since 1990.

Acknowledgements

With thanks to Brenda Cooper, Senior Lecturer in the Faculty of Health and Social Care, London South Bank University, for her helpful feedback on early material for this book.

Thanks also to my students who, over the years, have helped me refine and add to my understanding of this topic area.

Guide to the companion website accompanying this book

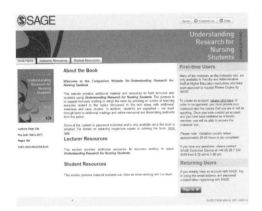

The companion website that accompanies this book provides students and lecturers with ready-to-use teaching and learning resources. They are free of charge and are designed to maximise the learning experience.

www.sagepub.co.uk/
ellis_research2e

For lecturers

Password protected material to ensure that only lecturers can access these resources. Registration is easy; just click on 'Lecturer Material' and if you have adopted the book, simply request a username and password from the email address supplied and access will be granted.

Extra activities and case studies

The author has provided some fantastic activities within the book that help to cement learning and encourage deeper understanding. We have taken this further by making extra materials available to provide a wider range of activities and case studies from all branches of nursing. These are downloadable and can be integrated into your VLE.

Powerpoint slides

The author has produced powerpoint slides to accompany each chapter that can be used within teaching or as handouts for students.

For students

Further reading and weblinks

There is a huge amount of information about nursing research available on the internet and knowing where to start is not easy. The author has helped by providing a manageable list of some fantastic websites that you would be wise to look at.

Podcasts from the author

If you want to study on the go or get some extra insight into the world of research, then why not listen to the podcasts prepared by the author that help to draw out some of the common challenges faced by students approaching this for the first time?

Introduction

The purpose of this book is to introduce the nursing student to the key concepts involved in nursing and healthcare research. The aim of introducing research is twofold: the first is to enable you to better understand the research you read to inform your practice and to make some judgements about its quality. The second reason is to prepare you to undertake research either as part of your role at work or as part of a course of study. Many nurses believe that understanding research, let alone undertaking research, is beyond them. This book sets out to explode this myth by demonstrating that the processes involved in the design and undertaking of research are easily understood.

Understanding Research for Nursing Students does not contain all that any budding researcher will need in order to design and carry out their own research, but it does provide a reasonable overview and suggests other sources of information that may help in the study design process. Clearly, books such as this present an idealistic view of research which is, like clinical nursing, subject to practical considerations and the realities of funding, experience and ability, and so rarely proceeds in a textbook manner.

Chapter 1 introduces what research in health and social care is about, and the sorts of questions that nursing research can be used to answer. It also introduces some of the philosophical assumptions that underpin research, including those that inform the quantitative and qualitative paradigms. The reader is introduced to the processes that a researcher might go through in order to generate a research question. In addition, Chapter 1 introduces the key ethical principles and ideas that inform all phases of the research process. It is important for any researcher to understand and take heed of these issues in the design of a research study in order to design a study that is both realistic and ethical.

Chapters 2 and 3 introduce qualitative research methodologies and methods. Chapter 2 concentrates on identifying the qualitative research methodologies, the questions they set out to answer, the sampling methods they use and the key methods (data collection tools) they employ. Chapter 3 continues the qualitative theme, exploring in more detail the key methods used in qualitative data collection. It goes on to explore some of the issues in data management and analysis of qualitative data.

Chapters 4 and 5 explore the quantitative research methodologies and some research methods. Chapter 4 mirrors Chapter 2 in introducing the quantitative research methodologies, the research questions they set out to answer, the ways in which samples for study are chosen and the key data collection methods they use. Chapter 4 concludes by introducing some of the key methods in data presentation and analysis used in the quantitative research methodologies. Chapter 5 continues to explore the quantitative theme, presenting some of the main methods nurses use when employing the quantitative methods in their research studies.

Chapter 6 examines the use of mixed methods and methodologies in research. It introduces the key ideas in evaluation research and the nature, scope and practice of action research in nursing, including data collection methods. This chapter establishes that there is often a need to employ mixed methodologies and methods in healthcare research in order to gain a more holistic view of some of the complex issues that surround the provision of nursing care.

This second edition of the book contains an additional short chapter about the thoughtful use of research to inform both what you do as a student nurse in practice and how research might be assimilated into your academic work to add to its depth and credibility. Chapter 7 demonstrates that research is not a dry academic topic but one potential source of increased knowledge to guide thinking and nursing practice.

NMC *Standards for Pre-registration Nursing Education* and Essential Skills Clusters

The Nursing and Midwifery Council (NMC) has standards of competence that have to be met by applicants to different parts of the nursing and midwifery register. These standards are what they deem as being necessary for the delivery of safe, effective nursing and midwifery practice.

As well as specific competencies, the NMC identifies specific skills nursing students must have at various points of their training programme. These Essential Skills Clusters (ESCs) are essential abilities that students need to attain in order to practise to their full potential.

This book identifies some of the competencies and skills within the realm of research and evidence-based practice, which student nurses need in order to be entered on to the NMC register. These competencies and ESCs are presented at the start of each chapter so that it is clear which of them the chapter addresses. All of the competencies and ESCs in this book relate to the *generic standards* which all nursing students must achieve. This book includes the latest NMC standards for 2010 onwards, taken from the *Standards for pre-registration nursing education* (NMC, 2010). For links to the pre-2010 standards, please visit the website for the book at www.learning matters.co.uk/nursing.

Learning features

Learning from reading text is not always easy. Therefore, to provide variety and to assist with the development of independent learning skills and the application of theory to practice, this book contains activities, case studies, concept summaries, further reading and useful websites to enable you to participate in your own learning. You will need to develop your own study skills and 'learn how to learn' to get the best from the material. The book cannot provide all the answers, but instead provides a framework for your learning.

The activities in the book will help you in particular to make sense of, and learn about, the material being presented. Some activities ask you to reflect on aspects of practice, or your experience of it, or the people or situations you encounter. *Reflection* is an essential skill in nursing, and it helps you to understand the world around you and often to identify how things might be improved. Other activities will help you develop key graduate skills such as your ability to *think critically* about a topic in order to challenge received wisdom, or your ability to *research a topic and find appropriate information and evidence*, and to be able to make decisions using that evidence in situations that are often difficult and time-pressured. Communication and working as part of a team are core to all nursing practice, and some activities will ask you to think about your *communication skills* to help develop these.

All the activities require you to take a break from reading the text, think through the issues presented and carry out some independent study, possibly using the internet. Where appropriate, there are sample answers presented at the end of each chapter, and these will help you to understand more fully your own reflections and independent study. You will gain most from the activities if you try to complete them yourself before reading the suggested answers. Remember, academic study will always require independent work; attending lectures will never be enough to be successful on your programme, and these activities will help to deepen your knowledge and understanding of the issues under scrutiny and give you practice at working on your own.

You might want to think about completing these activities as part of your personal development plan (PDP) or portfolio. After completing the activity write it up in your PDP or portfolio in a section devoted to that particular skill, then look back over time to see how far you have developed. You can also do more of the activities for a key skill that you have identified a weakness in, which will help build your skill and confidence in this area.

There is a glossary of terms at the end of the book that provides an interpretation of some of the terminology in the context of the subject of the book. Glossary terms are in **bold** in the first instance that they appear.

All chapters have further reading and useful websites listed at the end, with notes to show you why we think they will be helpful to you. The websites will also help you to remain up to date with developments in this aspect of practice as awareness of key issues grows and policies develop.

As well as an additional chapter this second edition of *Understanding Research for Nursing Students* has other improvements made in response to feedback from the earlier edition. These improvements include: more examples drawn from the various branches of nursing; the addition of more case studies; and an improved section on research statistics and research sampling.

Since the first edition there have been other research books written and published as well as additions and changes to existing websites, and these are reflected within this edition.

Most excitingly there are now some companion web pages to accompany this book. It is hoped this new facility will add to both your enjoyment and understanding of this topic area.

We hope that you find this book helpful in developing your professional practice and that it challenges you to ensure you provide care and support that reduces the risk of vulnerability and promotes dignity, respect and a positive quality of life. Good luck with your studies!

Chapter 1
Introducing research

NMC Standards for Pre-registration Nursing Education

This chapter will address the following competencies:

Domain 1: Professional values

7. All nurses must be responsible and accountable for keeping their knowledge and skills up to date through continuing professional development. They must aim to improve their performance and enhance the safety and quality of care through evaluation, supervision and appraisal.

9. All nurses must appreciate the value of evidence in practice, be able to understand and appraise research, apply relevant theory and research findings to their work, and identify areas for further investigation.

Domain 3: Nursing practice and decision making

10. All nurses must evaluate their care to improve clinical decision-making, quality and outcomes, using a range of methods, amending the plan of care, where necessary, and communicating changes to others.

Domain 4: Leadership, management and team working

6. All nurses must work independently as well as in teams. They must be able to take the lead in coordinating, delegating and supervising care safely, managing risk and remaining accountable for the care given.

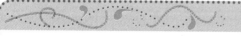

NMC Essential Skills Clusters

This chapter will address the following ESCs:

Organisational aspects of care

9. People can trust the newly registered graduate nurse to treat them as partners and work with them to make a holistic and systematic assessment of their needs; to develop a personalised plan that is based on mutual understanding and respect for their individual situation promoting health and well-being, minimising risk of harm and promoting their safety at all times.

For entry to the register:

14. Applies research based evidence to practice.

> ## Chapter aims
>
> After reading this chapter, you will be able to:
>
> - describe the nature of research in health and social care;
> - describe the type of questions that health and social care research is used to address;
> - demonstrate awareness of the philosophical underpinning of research;
> - describe the ethical considerations that need to be taken account of in health and social care research.

Introduction

The human condition is such that we are always striving to better ourselves and our lives. This is especially true of healthcare, where much money is invested each year in research and development. Many nurses think that research is something that is beyond them, something other people do, and that what they should do is simply respond by adopting new working practices following critical appraisal of the research. Unfortunately, recent practical, political and ethical restrictions on the undertaking of research by undergraduate and pre-registration healthcare professionals mean that this is indeed the case, and many nurses will never have the opportunity to experience the wonder of being the first to understand something or of discovering a new truth.

The truth about people who do research in nursing is not that they are different or in some way better than other nurses; it is more the fact that they have learned to ask questions about healthcare provision. Furthermore, they have learned to ask questions in very specific ways, ways that allow for the question to be explored and in some instances answered in a meaningful way. The purpose of this book is not to create world-class nurse researchers but to introduce you to the **methodologies** and **methods** that nursing and other healthcare researchers use to explore the exciting and challenging world of healthcare provision.

Before going any further, let us pause for a moment to think about what is meant by research in the context of this book. The term 'research' is used to describe the structured and conscious application of scientific method to the exploration of an issue of interest in order either to better understand the issue or to establish new truths. This process of understanding or establishing new truths is termed **empirical** research. Empiricist philosophers throughout the centuries have been concerned with establishing and understanding the nature of reality. So empirical research implies rather more than looking up a topic in the library or on the internet and discovering knowledge that is new to you. Empirical research is about discovering new knowledge and understanding for human kind.

Over the next five chapters, this book will take you on a tour of the major methodologies, methods and analytical processes used in nursing, health and social care research. The aim is to equip you with the understanding that will enable you not only to read and understand research in this area but also to think about how and why research is important to what we do as nurses. The book will establish what constitutes an appropriate research question, how research is undertaken, where and with whom research is undertaken, and what it can reasonably answer.

The research process

Coming up with a research question and then designing, undertaking, analysing and reporting research is a structured procedure that almost invariably follows the same process (see box below). This **research process** aids in ensuring that the research undertaken is fit for purpose; that is, it addresses the issue under consideration in a methodical manner.

The stages of the research process

- Identification of the issue in need of research (often a clinical issue).
- Undertaking a literature review (this stage is omitted in some qualitative methodologies).
- Stating the purpose of the research (what is it trying to achieve).
- Deciding the specific research questions, aims, objectives or hypotheses.
- Collecting the data.
- Analysing and interpreting the data.
- Evaluating and reporting the research findings.

The identification of a topic for research will more often than not be a response to a clinical or practice-related requirement. Such questions might arise out of uncertainty about what to do or what might work best for a given situation (see the following section on the uncertainty principle). In turn this uncertainty leads the researcher to the need to review the literature existing in a given area with the express purpose of deciding what it is the research can reasonably be expected to answer (this will depend on the nature of the question being asked (see the section on research paradigms on pages 11–12).

The nature of the problem being addressed will then determine the way in which the research question is asked. Since different methods are used to answer types of research questions, data collection will be determined not by researcher preference but in response to the need to use the right method to answer any given question. For example, if a question is about the handwashing behaviours of staff, the data collection method will need to include some element of observation, while if the question relates to staff understanding of the need for handwashing, then staff understanding can only be measured using questionnaires or interviews.

Once data are collected the analysis of the data needs to be driven by the type of data collected for the study, so data that are in numerical form will require statistical analysis and those in word form will need some form of **qualitative** data analysis. All research should then be subjected to some consideration of how well it has answered the original research question: Was it able to answer the question? Were there issues with the process that might be improved? Do the findings reflect other research in the area?

All of these elements of the research process will be addressed in more detail in the subsequent sections of this chapter and in more specific detail within the various chapters of this book.

The uncertainty principle

The starting point for all research is uncertainty. Uncertainty in the case of research is no bad thing. It is the lack of certainty in an area that creates a question. Uncertainty arises in all areas of health and social care, from questioning whether a new drug will cure cancer to understanding what it is like to live with respiratory disease.

Concept summary: the uncertainty principle

The **uncertainty principle** is the starting point for all research, as it establishes that there is something about the care we provide that we are not sure of. We may be uncertain how patients make sense of living with a disease, or how they understand the care we are providing, or indeed whether the care we provide is beneficial to them. Uncertainty causes us to ask questions. If we take the examples above and apply them to specific care scenarios, some questions we might ask are:

- what is it like to live with multiple sclerosis?
- do patients undergoing chemotherapy understand its purpose?
- does daily dressing of pressure ulcers aid their healing?
- what are the mental health issues facing individuals with learning disabilities?

Each of these scenarios is important in different ways, and each leads us to ask questions about what we do as nurses; each contains an element of uncertainty.

So if the starting point for research is uncertainty, where do we move to next? Plainly there is a need to frame research questions that are relevant to the problem being considered, and that are also able to address the uncertainty raised. It is important here to state that, because of the element of uncertainty that underlies each question, there is also uncertainty about whether the question we pose can be answered satisfactorily. So at the heart of research lies uncertainty not only about an element of care but also about how, and indeed whether, we can actually answer the questions raised. Research seeks to answer questions, but there are no guarantees that it can.

Why is research important then? If we cannot guarantee that research can answer the questions we pose, why do it? These are very reasonable questions. Any research is only as good as the methodologies and methods it employs. All research methodologies and methods have their strengths and weaknesses, and all research findings are open to being disproved or modified by later research. What is important about nursing research is that researchers try to answer, to the best of their ability, important questions about the care we give.

Using research to answer questions about the care we give is important because it allows us to develop increasing certainty about what we do. It allows us, as nurses, to be able to justify our practice; it provides, at least in part, an evidence base.

Activity 1.1   *Critical thinking*

Make a list of the reasons, both clinical and political, why research is important in informing the practice of nurses. Don't think just about the individual patient, think also about wider society and the greater good.

An outline answer of what you might find is given at the end of the chapter.

Developing research questions

So far we have seen that the starting point for research is uncertainty about a question or questions that, in the context of this book at least, arise out of clinical practice. How, then, do we ask questions and what structures might we apply to the process?

Asking questions for research requires considerable thought, not only about the question itself but about whether the answer to our questions already exists. It may be that the questions arise out of clinical observations or interactions that have occurred in practice. Such questions may lead us down one of two pathways. The first is to seek clarification of the state of knowledge by reading the existing literature within the area of interest. The second is to ask questions that as yet have no, or only limited, answers.

Reviewing the literature on a topic is in itself a skill and one with which you may already be familiar. The existence of high quality, readily accessible bibliographic databases makes it increasingly easy to scrutinise the literature in order to find out the state of knowledge in a particular area. Online databases, such as the Cumulative Index of Nursing and Allied Health Literature (CINAHL), are a first point of call for many researchers. It is worth taking time and making the effort to learn and understand the processes by which these databases can be searched. Your university or hospital librarian will most certainly be able to help with this.

It is important to realise that, even if research has already been carried out within a given area, there may still be questions about its applicability to particular situations or circumstances. Gomm (2000a and 2000b) asks two important questions of research: 'Would it work here?' and 'Should we afford it?' Gomm points out that just because research has shown that a certain intervention works in one setting with a particular set of individuals does not mean that it will work somewhere else. For instance, because a particular health education programme has worked in England among older people with hypertension does not mean that it will work in India, or among younger people, or indeed among people who have another disease entirely.

'Should we afford it?' (Gomm, 2000b) makes the point that some interventions in the health and social care setting may be so expensive and their benefits so minimal that it may not be appropriate to use them. Indeed, we may, in the process of reviewing the literature, identify other, less costly, interventions that provide a similar, or equal, level of benefit. Quite clearly there are also ethical and moral questions about what level and types of heath care interventions society should fund.

Gaining answers to these questions is important both when searching the literature and in planning research. Having answers to both these questions helps the would-be researcher decide whether what they want to do is of potential benefit. The whole purpose of research in nursing is that it provides us with knowledge to improve what we do and how we do it.

Once the research literature has been searched and a need for further research to answer a question of importance to practice has been identified, the researcher will move on to formulating a question that will guide the design and execution of the research project.

There are two models for question formulation that are widely used in health and social research. These models allow the researcher to focus not only on the research question but also on how the literature databases will be searched. Each model employs an acronym (SPICE and PICO) that helps the researcher focus and frame the research question in a logical and methodical manner.

The SPICE model is most commonly applied to research aimed at answering questions that have a qualitative element to them (see later). SPICE stands for:

- Setting;
- Perspective;
- Intervention;
- Comparison;
- Evaluation.

A couple of examples of the application of the SPICE model will help to illustrate how it helps to frame the search and research question. In our first example, we want to explore patients' understanding of living with asthma. We choose to focus on patients who are not usually unwell as a result of their asthma, and so concentrate on the general practice *setting*. The *perspective* of the study, i.e. what the research is about, is clearly asthma. Because we are interested in people's understanding, we will not be applying an *intervention*. *Comparisons* of understanding might arise, possibly by chance, from the study, for instance between those newly diagnosed and those with a long-established diagnosis. The *evaluation* of the study will involve understanding people's perceptions of living with asthma and exploring these perceptions.

Activity 1.2   *Critical thinking*

Using the SPICE model, decide how you might frame a research question relating to a problem or issue from your area of practice. Remember, it is not necessary to use all of the elements of the models in every type of research. Which of the elements you use will depend on the type of question you are asking.

As the answer is based on your own observation, there is no outline answer at the end of the chapter.

In our second example we are interested in the effects of an education programme on people's understanding of living with asthma. Our *setting* is again general practice. Our *perspective* remains asthma. Because we want to measure the effects of the education programme, we clearly are applying an *intervention*, which is the education programme. In order to understand the effectiveness of the programme, we need something to *compare* to. This might be people's understanding of asthma before and after the programme or it might be the difference in understanding between one group who had the intervention and another group who did not. Our *evaluation* will then consist of identifying the level of difference in understanding between the intervention and non-intervention groups.

The PICO model is usually applied to research studies that involve an intervention, although, as we have seen, the SPICE model can also be used for this purpose. PICO stands for:

- Patient or Problem;
- Intervention;
- Comparison;
- Outcome.

PICO will work equally well as a method of illuminating the elements of the second example above. In this instance, therefore, *patient* refers to patients in general practice with asthma. The *intervention* remains the education programme. *Comparison* is still that of understanding before and after the education programme, while *outcome* refers to the improvement, or not, in patients' understanding of living with asthma.

Activity 1.3   *Critical thinking*

Using the PICO model, decide how you might frame a research question relating to a problem or issue from your area of practice. Remember, it is not necessary to use all of the elements of the models in every type of research. Which of the elements you use will depend on the type of question you are asking.

As the answer is based on your own observation, there is no outline answer at the end of the chapter.

Once framed in this way, it is easier to create a list of all the words and phrases associated with the potential research question. This list will itself enable you to structure your literature review, which will in turn inform the research plan. Such a list will include not only the key words but also synonyms, and lay and technical terminology. For example, pressure ulcers may appear as pressure sores, decubitus ulcers, bed sores, skin ulcers, etc. It would be useful to search using all of these terms.

It is also helpful to apply some limits within which the bibliographic database should search: for example, it may be helpful to limit the search to the last five or ten years depending on the topic. It is also worth asking your hospital or university librarian about access to other sources of information such as unpublished reports or university theses.

The literature search and identification of existing research is likely to leave you in one of three positions. The first is that the topic that you are interested in has already been well researched, and the research covers a similar patient group to the one you care for. Depending on the age of the research, you may feel further research to inform a potential change in practice is unnecessary. However, it is always worth being cautious about applying research that has only been undertaken once without putting in place some form of local evaluation and audit of the change. This is because sometimes research can actually come to the wrong conclusions!

The second position is that the research has been done, but in a group, or in a place, very dissimilar to where you want to apply it. For example, the research may have been done abroad, the ages of the participants may be very different from the patients that you care for or the patients may have come from a different ethnic or cultural background. This may lead you back to Gomm's (2000a) question, 'Would it work here?'

The third situation is that the research has not been done anywhere that you can find. So you are left where you started, with a question, or questions, that need answering. It is important to look at these questions and identify approaches that might usefully be employed in answering them. At this point, it might be useful to return to your PICO or SPICE model in order to help you think about how to structure and present the research question.

Before we go on to explore how we place our question within a research framework, a note of caution is needed. Some research, such as grounded theory and phenomenology (explained in Chapter 2), requires researchers to start with limited preconceptions about what they might find. This means that it may be necessary for a researcher to avoid engaging in a full literature search at the start of the study. This is something that should be discussed with a research supervisor.

You may have noticed that the questions we have asked so far fall into two distinct categories. The first category includes questions about things we can measure directly, such as the rate of healing of a pressure ulcer. The second category is more elusive. It is about feelings, understanding and being, and is therefore more difficult to measure in any direct, objective way.

Research paradigms

This difference in the emphasis of the questions asked leads us to the first rung of the research ladder: identifying the nature of the question being asked. In research terminology this means we need to identify the **paradigm** within which the question sits. Simply put, paradigms are the philosophical basis of the question being asked, the nature of the enquiry needed in order to address the question that has been identified.

In health and social care research, as in most practical research, it is usual to identify two paradigms, the **quantitative paradigm** and the **qualitative paradigm**. These paradigms refer to two different ways of viewing the world and reality.

The quantitative paradigm is perhaps the one you might most associate with scientific ways of thinking and enquiry. It involves viewing the world in ways that are measurable – provable if you like. The 'quantitative' element of the paradigm refers to the ability of research within this paradigm to quantify its findings. In other words, the findings can be counted or can be demonstrated in a way that is measurable.

Quantitative research is concerned with proof, with cause and effect and with demonstrating associations between **variables**. Quantitative research often starts with a **hypothesis**, an idea yet to be tested using established scientific methods. Chapter 4 explores the approaches to research that lie within this research paradigm.

Activity 1.4   *Reflection*

Given that quantitative research paradigms are concerned with things that can be counted, and with cause and effect, think about what questions you could ask about where you currently work that fit this paradigm. What clinical problems might be best answered using this approach?

Keep your notes on this safe and return to them when you read Chapter 4 where you will find many examples of this type of research to compare your notes to.

Data collection within the quantitative paradigm is **deductive**. That is, quantitative research starts with a hypothesis, or idea, that it seeks to confirm or refute. Deductive reasoning follows predetermined methods for collecting data. Deductive research works from general observations towards a more specific outcome and in this respect it is considered to be 'knowledge driven' – that is, it is about things we think we know, such as things we see and things we can quantify. Its primary purpose is to prove or disprove areas of perceived knowledge. Figure 1.1 gives a diagrammatic representation of deductive research.

The qualitative paradigm is the one that you might most associate with the social sciences and 'people-centred' methods of enquiry. It is a way of looking at the world from the point of view of people. It enquires about what people feel, think, understand and believe. The qualitative paradigm is not so concerned with proof – more with describing and understanding human experiences from the point of view of the people who have had, or are having, the experience.

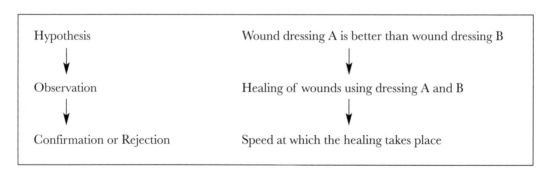

Figure 1.1: Representation of deductive research

The 'qualitative' element of the paradigm refers to the fact that it seeks to understand things that cannot readily be measured or counted. It is more concerned with the quality of an experience and of understanding and belief. Qualitative research starts with a question, something that needs to be explored; it may be used to generate a hypothesis, but it does not start with one. Chapter 2 explores the approaches to enquiry used within this paradigm.

Activity 1.5 — *Reflection*

Given that the qualitative research paradigm is concerned with things that cannot be counted, such as human experiences and understanding, think about what questions you could ask about where you currently work that fit this paradigm. What clinical problems might be best answered using this approach?

Keep your notes on this safe and return to them in Chapter 2 where you will find many examples of this type of research to which you can compare your answer.

Qualitative research is by its very nature **inductive**. That is, it generates ideas and theories from what is observed during the research. The data collected lead to the generation of ideas or hypotheses (hypotheses tested in deductive studies, as discussed above, are sometimes derived from inductive research). The researchers start out on an enquiry not knowing what they will find; they allow the data collected to lead them to the creation of a new idea or hypothesis. Inductive research works from specific observations towards creating much broader generalisations. Sometimes described as 'feature detecting', it uses observations and interviews to detect the key features of a phenomenon. Figure 1.2 gives a diagrammatic representation of inductive research.

It is worth reflecting on the generic competency introduced at the start of this chapter that requires nurses to practise autonomously, applying 'relevant theory and research' to practice. This assumes that the nurse has an understanding of the theoretical basis of research and the variety and types of questions that research can be used to answer. Even at this stage of the book, you

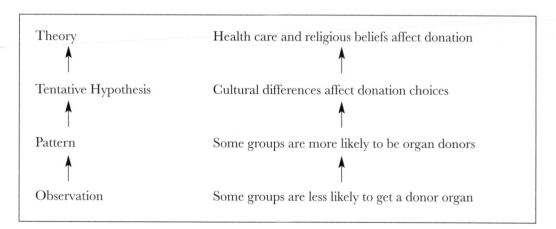

Figure 1.2: Representation of inductive research

should already be in a position to identify that there are two main research approaches (or paradigms) that inform the ways in which information for practice is generated. You may, as an individual, have a particular preference for one type of questioning over the other. If you do, how does this preference affect your interactions in the clinical setting?

We have established that there are two key routes to understanding the world of healthcare using the qualitative and quantitative paradigms. Now it is important that we identify how these apparently opposing world views are put into practice to answer research questions that arise in the clinical setting.

Within each paradigm there are a number of approaches to research that are used to answer specific types of questions. These approaches to research are called research methodologies, a term we used above. The following section of this chapter will introduce you to the key elements of the research methodologies that will be explored in more depth in Chapters 2 and 4.

Research methodologies

If the research paradigms are the schools of thought upon which research is based, the methodologies represent the more detailed plan of action used to execute the research. The term 'methodology' refers to the blueprint for action upon which an enquiry is based. Methodologies supply structure to the research process as they are designed to be undertaken in specific ways in order to answer specific questions.

Examples of the use of a methodology within a paradigm include **randomised controlled trials**, which seek to prove cause and effect and so sit within the quantitative paradigm, and **phenomenology,** which explores people's experiences of a phenomenon and so sits within the qualitative paradigm. Table 1.1 shows the research paradigms and the major research methodologies that are explored in this book. This is not an exhaustive list, and, as we shall see at various points in the book and especially in Chapter 6, clinical questions often generate the need for research to operate in more than one paradigm.

Research methodologies are, therefore, the overall scheme by which research is undertaken, and the choice of methodology is driven by the nature of this research question being asked.

We now know that the broad research question determines the paradigm within which a research approach lies and that the specific question will then determine the methodology to be applied. Chapters 2 and 4 will examine in more detail how these choices are made and why.

Table 1.1: The research paradigms and their major associated methodologies

Research paradigm	*Qualitative paradigm*	*Quantitative paradigm*
Research methodologies	Phenomenology	Randomised controlled trial
	Grounded theory	Cohort study
	Ethnography	Case-control studies
	Case study	Cross-sectional studies

Once the methodology has been decided upon, the exact methods, or tools, for data collection can be chosen.

Research methods

Research methods are the tools by which the information for an enquiry is collected. They are the practical equipment used to gather the data for the study. The choice of paradigm and subsequent research methodology will determine which research methods are used in an enquiry.

Clearly, the methods of data collection have to fit the type of question asked. For example, if the research is about understanding how people feel, how they see the world or how they see their experiences, then the researcher needs to ask them about these things. Such an enquiry requires the researcher to engage in dialogue with the research subjects, using interviews, focus groups or observation in order to gain an insight into their world. These issues cannot be measured or quantified in any meaningful way, so these qualitative methods allow an insight into someone else's world that cannot be gained using quantitative methodologies.

Conversely, it is not possible to demonstrate that a new wound dressing has some additional clinical benefit for patients by talking to them. Such things need to be measured, and a level of comparison between the new dressing and some existing dressing needs to be undertaken. In order to undertake such an enquiry, the researcher will need to take some biological and clinical measurements that can be enumerated. For example, how long does the wound take to heal? How many days does the patient spend in hospital? These are questions that cannot be addressed meaningfully, or accurately, by qualitative methodologies.

So far, we have established that research generally falls into one of two paradigms, although (as we will see in this book) some research questions may require a blend of the two approaches in order to answer them satisfactorily. We have identified that certain methodologies are associated with each of the two paradigms and that, within the methodologies, certain methods are used to collect the data for the study.

As well as thinking about and selecting the best methodology and methods for a study there are other considerations that a researcher has to take into account when designing and undertaking a study. Some of these will be explored in the following sections of the chapter.

Activity 1.6   *Research and finding out*

Before proceeding to read the rest of the chapter, make some notes about what other things a researcher might need to take into account when designing a study.

An outline of what you might find is given at the end of the chapter.

Ethical considerations in research

Ethics permeate all that we do in the delivery of health and social care. It is a requirement of nursing practice that we act in ways that are ethical and that take into account the rights of the people we care for (see the competency cited at the beginning of this chapter for the 'Leadership, management and team working' domain of the Nursing and Midwifery Council's (NMC) competency framework, as well as the NMC's *Code of Professional Conduct*, 2008). Ethical considerations in research are important for many reasons, not least of which is that people enter into research studies of their own free will (unlike entering hospital when unwell, for example) and that the research that we are undertaking is premised on the fact that we do not know what we will find – the uncertainty principle.

It is a sad fact of life that some of the clinical information we use today in healthcare provision has been obtained at the expense of the weak and vulnerable in society. Immediate examples that spring to mind are the atrocities committed by Nazi doctors in the name of medical research in the concentration and extermination camps of the Second World War. But there are also many more recent examples of unethical and immoral practices in healthcare, within societies considered to be world leaders in the promotion and protection of human rights.

Case study

'The Tuskegee Study of Untreated Syphilis in the Negro Male' was a clinical study of the effects of syphilis conducted over the 40 years between 1932 and 1972 in Tuskegee, Alabama, in the United States of America. A total of 399 male African Americans infected with syphilis were enrolled in the study along with a control group of 201 (people without syphilis). All of the participants were poor, most were illiterate and they did not give informed consent. They were not told about their diagnosis; rather, they were told they had 'bad blood' and would get taken to the clinic to receive free medical treatment, as well as free meals and burial insurance, as incentives for participating.

*When the study started, existing treatments for syphilis were often toxic and of limited, if any, effectiveness. One of the initial aims of the study was to establish whether patients were better off not being treated with these dubious remedies. Many participants were therefore denied any treatment, and others were lied to and given **placebo** (fake) treatments so that the fatal progression of the syphilis could be observed.*

At the end of the study, only 74 of the participants were still alive; 28 had died of syphilis while 100 died of syphilis-related complications. As well as the effects on the study subjects, 40 wives had become infected, and 19 of their children had been born with congenital syphilis.

The Declaration of Helsinki

Such instances, as well as other notoriously unethically conducted studies, led to the establishment of various conventions and international agreements on the ethical conduct of research involving human subjects. Perhaps the most widely known of these is the Declaration of Helsinki, first published by the World Medical Association in 1964 and most recently revised in 2008 (World Medical Association, 2008). There are three key tenets of the declaration of Helsinki.

- Studies should be of a generally acceptable scientific standard.
- The study should cause no harm.
- The study subjects should have given their full consent.

What these mean for the various stages of the research process depends upon interpretation and the type of research being undertaken. Before exploring in a little more detail the application of ethics to research, it is worth considering what approaches to ethics might be used to inform that process.

Approaches to ethics

Beauchamp and Childress (2008) present the ethical principles of **beneficence** (doing good), **non-maleficence** (doing no harm), **autonomy** (respecting choice) and **justice** (fairness) as one way of viewing the moral and ethical obligations of human beings. These principles may equally well be applied to research being undertaken in the human setting.

These are duty-based ethical principles that identify the individual human being as the central point of importance in ethical thinking, and dictate the way in which researchers should behave towards their study participants. This duty-based (or **non-consequentialist**) approach requires researchers to follow certain rules of conduct regardless of their consequences. This way of thinking about ethics has strong associations with both Judaism and Christianity, as it is based on the standards of human behaviour dictated by the Ten Commandments.

In contrast to duty-based ethics, **utilitarian** (or **consequentialist**) ethics take the view that the ends justify the means – that is, the consequence of the action is more important than the action undertaken. So consequentialist ethics require us to make a judgement about the likely outcome of a course of action, whereas duty-based ethics require us always to act in a way that is in itself good.

We have seen that uncertainty is the starting point for all research, and so it might seem impossible to apply these principles to the research process precisely because we cannot be certain how the research will proceed and what its consequences might be. It is important, however, to take the view that ethics are as much about intentions as they are about what actually happens. Given that the research has the right intentions, and that some of the basic principles of ethics, such as avoiding doing unnecessary harm and aiming for a good outcome, are followed, it is possible to undertake research in an ethical way.

For the researcher setting out to undertake an enquiry, and for the practising nurse who is reading the results of the research and seeking to use them in their day-to-day practice, it is important that the ethics of each stage of the research process are well established. Most, if not all, nursing, medical and health journals now require that all research papers submitted for publication can show that they have received ethics committee approval.

Ethics in the stages of research

The first stage of the research process is deciding what we are going to research and how. Certainly there are ethical issues to be addressed here, including whether the potential benefits of the study are great enough to justify the time, money and effort that will be used in undertaking it. Because we cannot know for certain about the answers to any of these issues, we have to ask questions about the intentions of the study. If the intention of the study is to improve the lives of future patients and clients, then it is reasonable to move to the next question.

The second question that arises is whether or not the study will inflict harm on the research subjects. Again we cannot know for certain whether or not this will happen. Even qualitative enquiries, which involve little more than an interview or a focus group discussion, have the potential to upset people – for example, by encouraging them to confront thoughts and feelings they had suppressed. It is important, therefore, that if the effects of the study cannot be known before the study starts, there should at least be mechanisms in place to minimise any harm that does arise. In a qualitative study this might mean providing counselling or support services for participants. Making such provisions satisfies the requirements of avoiding deliberate harm as well as attaining the best consequences for research participants by minimising unforeseen and unintended consequences of the study.

If the study is likely to inflict some harm, as may be the case in a drug trial or a study of a new surgical procedure, we may wish to ask whether or not the likely outcomes of the study make the potential for harm worthwhile. This is not a decision to be taken lightly. It is necessary for all research to be designed in a way that minimises the likelihood of this occurring – that it is of a generally acceptable scientific standard (World Medical Association, 2008). Any risks, or potential risks, associated with a study need to be disclosed at the point of gaining consent, so that whether the risk is worth taking is a decision that potential participants can make for themselves.

Gaining consent

Gaining consent from potential research participants is not a one-off event. The gaining and maintenance of consent is regarded as an ongoing process by the NHS National Research Ethics Service (NRES, 2008) and the NMC (2008). Gaining true and valid consent for any study may appear impossible given the fact that the outcome of the research is not known at the point that the consent is gained! This should not impede the process of research, nor should it be thought that it makes the process of gaining consent fraudulent. Consent gained in relation to a piece of research is for the participation of the individual in a process that will lead to an as yet uncertain outcome. Consent to participate in research has to be obtained in all cases and for all types of studies.

Consent can be described as a process that takes into account a number of separate elements:

- the competence of the potential participant to give their consent;
- the understanding of the information given;
- freedom from coercion;
- freedom of choice;
- the understanding of the right to withdraw.

Given the nature of health and social care research – the sort of research that nurses may become involved in – the research participants are likely to be in some way vulnerable (e.g. in poor health or elderly). This vulnerability leads to concerns about the competence of the individuals to consent. Such concerns include people who, when well, are without doubt competent.

It is clear that some individuals are not, and will never be, competent to give consent – for example, people with dementia and young children. In the UK the NRES provides clear guidance on what to do in situations where the consent of an individual cannot be gained because of their age or illness. This includes respecting previously given consent, or withheld consent, and seeking the consent of the next of kin or parents where appropriate (NRES, 2008).

Next, we have to ensure that the potential research participants for a study have received information about the study and understood it. This means producing information sheets that are written in a manner that potential participants can understand, checking that potential participants have understood and explaining any ambiguities or misunderstandings. It is at this stage that the help of lay collaborators in research can be invaluable.

Freedom from coercion means ensuring that potential participants do not feel under any obligation to take part in the study. Coercion may result from the fact that the potential participant and the researcher are in a dependent relationship. Such relationships, which might include nurse–patient or student–lecturer relationships, may make the potential participant feel under an obligation to take part in a study. In such cases, great care must be taken to ensure that potential research participants are aware that they are under no obligation to take part, and that not taking part will have no adverse effect on their care or education.

Freedom of choice means ensuring that potential participants understand that they are under no obligation to choose to take part in the study. The choice made should be one they enter into, having read and understood the information given to them and decided they want to participate. They must be free to choose not to participate if that is their wish.

Research participants should also understand they have the right to withdraw from a study at any point. This is what is meant by consent being an ongoing process. Just because an individual agrees to start a study does not mean that they have to see it through to the end against their wishes.

Confidentiality

A further key element of research ethics is the protection of the confidentiality of research participants. Any participant in a study has the right to expect that he or she will not be identifiable when the findings of the research are made public and that participation in research will not lead to any disadvantage for them. The advent of genetic diagnoses has made the issue of participant data confidentiality very topical. Participants are worried that data taken from their DNA for research purposes could lead to increased insurance premiums should it be shown to suggest that they have a high risk of developing a genetically determined disease.

Aside from these 'high tech' studies, people involved in studies in which they express controversial opinions or disclose personal information about their battle with disease may wish for the source of this information to be kept private. It is therefore incumbent on the ethical researcher to adhere to a strict code of confidentiality both while undertaking the research and when writing it up for publication or conference presentation.

Disseminating research

Right at the start of the research process we saw how important it was to look into the existing literature about a topic in order either to inform an immediate change in practice or to design a research study. This means that there is an ethical need for researchers to make the findings of their work public. Withholding the findings of research has consequences for other researchers, who may set out to undertake research into an area that has already been explored, using time and money that could be better spent elsewhere.

There are a number of reasons why not all studies get published. Sometimes the research is undertaken as part of a course of study, and the student, on getting their award, feels that they have completed all they need to do. Sometimes the research comes out with a result that was unexpected – it disproves the hypothesis, perhaps. This may lead some researchers not to publish, especially where the research has been sponsored by an organisation that may be damaged by the negative findings. Another reason that research with negative findings does not get published is that it is rejected by publishers because it does not make good reading.

If we return to our guiding ethical principles, we can say that not publishing or making the findings of research known is potentially unethical for two reasons: it may inflict harm on others and it may lead to negative consequences. The 'others' on which harm may be inflicted include: the people who volunteered for the study who expected their sacrifice to benefit other people; researchers who subsequently design studies that are in the same area or contain the same flaws that may have been identified had they seen the previous research; and people who are current patients who may be subjected to care that research has shown does not work.

Other issues to take into account when designing a research project

As well as the research question and the ethical issues, there are a number of things a potential researcher has to take into account before starting on a piece of research. Some of these issues will be discussed in the following paragraphs.

Even the simplest study will have some cost attached to it. Interviewing participants for a study may involve travel, the cost of the recording device and often the cost of professional transcription of the interview tapes. Other costs that may need to be considered, depending on the study, are postage, printing, and paperwork and telephone costs. Many novice researchers underestimate the time that a study will take to do and so may not cost out the time away from work that research grants are often designed to help with.

The amount of time needed to undertake research often comes as a surprise to the first-time researcher. Time needed for a study will include the time taken to read textbooks regarding research design as well as the time taken to undertake a literature review of the topic under research. The study will then need to be written up for ethical and, potentially, research and development review (that is, a review of the scientific quality of the study as well as what the study may mean in terms of the use of facilities and staff time within the organisation within which it is set). There is a need to write participant literature, undertake the data collection (whatever form that takes), review and analyse the data and then write the study up. Interestingly, the time taken to prepare to undertake the study and the time taken to analyse the findings are both often far in excess of the time taken to actually do the study itself.

Even the most experienced researchers will rely to some extent on the expertise of others at some stage of the research process – most commonly at the study design stage and at the analysis stage. It is often worth getting advice about how the study will be analysed at the design stage in order to ensure that data that are collected are in the right format and of the best type to allow for the best possible analysis. Collecting the correct type of data in the correct format is most important in quantitative studies that will be subjected to statistical analysis, as some forms of data will increase the power of the study.

Because a study can take a long time to do, one of the issues that commonly affects the novice researcher is maintaining their interest, which can wane especially during the design and analysis stages. One of the questions the researcher must ask themselves at the start of any study is, therefore, 'Will this study hold my attention for its duration?'

Chapter summary

This chapter has introduced you to the key elements that need to be considered when setting out to undertake a research project. It has identified that in nursing, there are two broad approaches to answering clinical questions. These approaches – the quantitative and qualitative paradigms – have distinct features and may be used to answer specific types of questions. The choice of research paradigm is determined by the type of question the research seeks to answer, and it is important this is understood from the start of the research process.

We have seen that the choice of paradigm and the nature of the research question then leads the researcher to select an overall methodology – research approach – for their study. The methodology chosen determines the methods, or research tools, that the researcher will apply in undertaking the research.

The need to apply ethical considerations to all stages of the research process has been discussed, and ethical theories used to illustrate why this is important. Ethical considerations have been identified as being more important than scientific considerations when designing a research project.

This chapter has also identified some of the practical considerations potential researchers need to take into account before starting out on a research project. This is important for making sure time and money are spent wisely.

Activities: Brief outline answers

Activity 1.1: Critical thinking (page 8)

There are several reasons why research is important in informing nursing practice.

- It shows that we can account for our actions.
- It shows that what we do is ethical – it does good or at least avoids doing harm.
- It shows that we are spending public money wisely.
- It demonstrates that what we do is of clinical benefit.
- It responds to the need for governance.
- It establishes the professional credibility of nursing practice.

Activity 1.6: Research and finding out (page 15)

What a researcher might need to take into account when designing a study:

- their own expertise;
- money;
- the availability of time;
- ethical issues;
- access to research subjects;
- availability of support.

Further reading

Hek, G and Moule, P (2011) *Making sense of research: an introduction for health and social care practitioners* (4th edn). London: Sage.

Chapters 1 and 2 establish the need for and nature of research in the caring professions.

Parahoo, K (2006) *Nursing research: principles, process and issues* (2nd edn). London: Palgrave Macmillan.

Chapters 1 and 2 provide a good overview of the sources of and need for knowledge in nursing.

Topping, A (2010) The quantitative-qualitative continuum, in Gerish, K and Lacey, A (eds) *The research process in nursing* (6th edn). Oxford: Wiley-Blackwell.

A useful discussion of the nature of knowledge and qualitative and quantitative research paradigms.

Useful websites

www.niehs.nih.gov/research/resources/bioethics/whatis.cfm An overview of research ethics including case studies.

www.nres.nhs.uk/ UK NHS research ethics committee's website.

www.rcn.org.uk/__data/assets/pdf_file/0007/388591/003138.pdf The new RCN guidance on research ethics for nurses, which provides a useful overview of good practice.

www.rlo-cetl.ac.uk:8080/open_virtual_file_path/i2529n6682t/index.html An animated and spoken introduction to qualitative and quantitative research paradigms.

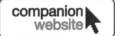

For further activities and other useful material, visit the companion website at **www.sagepub.co.uk/ellis_research2e**

Chapter 2
Overview of qualitative methodologies

Chapter aims

After reading this chapter, you will be able to:

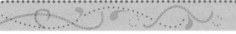

- identify the main qualitative research methodologies used in health and social care;
- describe the type of research questions the different qualitative research methodologies can be used to answer;
- demonstrate awareness of how samples are chosen for qualitative studies;
- briefly describe the key methods of data collection used in each methodology.

Introduction

In Chapter 1, it was established that qualitative research is research that answers questions about people's attitudes, experiences and opinions. Qualitative research differs from quantitative research in the way it approaches research questions. The key is in the name: quantitative research is concerned with quantity so uses numbers; qualitative research is concerned with the nature and quality of individuals' experience. The data used in qualitative research are words and sometimes pictures. Qualitative research is essentially expressive and people centred – that is, it is focused on people's lived experiences, attitudes, opinions and feelings.

Nursing is often described as both an art and a science. It is, perhaps, the art of nursing that qualitative research best addresses, as it answers questions not about the science of what we do as nurses but about the art of human interaction. At the same time, qualitative research tries to understand something of the lives of the people we care for. Nursing is a people-centred discipline, and qualitative research has found favour among nursing academics and practitioners because of its ability to ask and answer questions about what it is like to be someone else, what it is like to experience care and how people in receipt of care view that care.

As Table 2.1 shows, different kinds of qualitative research look at different forms of human interaction.

Table 2.1: The main qualitative research designs used in nursing

Research design	Usages
Phenomenology	Studies a phenomenon or experience of interest
Grounded theory	Generates a theory about a social interaction
Ethnography	Studies groups and cultures
Case study	Explores a case or a number of cases of interest
Generic qualitative	Follows the methods but does not identify a methodology

Key characteristics of qualitative research

Qualitative research is used to answer some of the questions that quantitative research cannot. For instance, we cannot measure someone's emotions or attitudes using a ruler or a thermometer, therefore we cannot quantify them – try as we might to create scales that measure this sort of data. Many questions that need answering about nursing and healthcare are not related to numbers of patients treated, the speed of recovery, time spent in hospital or mortality rates. Questions such as 'How well do I feel I have been cared for?' or 'What is it like to be treated in this dialysis unit?' are more about the perceived quality of the care provided than the actual amount.

Activity 2.1   *Critical thinking*

Next time you are working clinically, try asking one or more service users this simple question: 'What is it like to be treated here?' Make a note of the responses and spend some time reflecting on how the views reflected in the answers are different from your view of where you work.

As the answer will be based on your experience, there is no outline answer at the end of the chapter.

What is clear is that different people experience the same phenomenon in different ways. An understanding of how the care we give is experienced by those we care for will therefore be of benefit to nurses who are concerned with *how* they deliver care.

The radically different emphases of qualitative and quantitative questions, and the fact that they are both equally important to our understanding of care, means that there are a large number of differences not only in the philosophy underpinning each paradigm but also in the research methodologies and methods they use.

Some academics and researchers like to claim that one paradigm is more important, or indeed better, than the other. This view of research as being competitive in nature and differing in importance is really quite short-sighted. It is perhaps better to think about the two forms of research as being of equal importance, with the findings from one complementing and adding extra dimensions to the findings of the other.

Quite often quantitative research generates the need for an answer to a qualitative question. That is, sometimes we find out things by experiment or measurement that leave us with another, perhaps equally or more important, question. For example, Professor Sir Richard Doll famously demonstrated the link between smoking and lung cancer, using quantitative research, but people continue to smoke. An important question that arises from this for nursing practice in terms of a public health message is, therefore, 'Why do people smoke?' The answers to why people take up smoking and continue to smoke can only realistically be gained from an insight into the motivations, understandings and stories of people who smoke. Qualitative research methods are needed to gain this valuable understanding.

It is only if and when we can answer such important questions as 'Why do people smoke?' that we can address the next logical question, 'How can we stop people from smoking?' Of course, the answer to this question may partially lie within a quantitative question such as 'Is using nicotine replacement therapy better than not using it in helping people to quit smoking?' Or we may need to ask a question such as 'What do people say about what causes them to continue smoking when they know it is harming them?' – a qualitative enquiry.

The various qualitative methodologies have evolved to answer quite specific questions using often well-defined methods. For example, we will see that phenomenological research has developed to answer questions about the '**essence**', or 'meaning', of a particular experience, or phenomenon, and the method usually used to answer this type of question is in-depth interviewing.

It is quite common for qualitative studies to identify themselves simply as 'a qualitative study' when published and not to identify one specific methodology that informed the approach to answering the question. While, in this chapter, specific qualitative research methodologies are presented as being used to answer specific questions using well-defined and attached methods, it is not unreasonable for a qualitative researcher to adopt some of the methods of qualitative research in order to answer their research question without necessarily identifying and adopting a specific methodology.

At first glance this may seem odd; however, all experienced researchers know that in order to successfully undertake any research, compromises have to be made, and often established rules and conventions associated with a particular methodology may prove hard to follow in the pursuit of answering a specific qualitative question. The methods used and the processes adopted within the practice of qualitative research often evolve and develop during the life of the study in response to difficulties encountered or insights gained. This evolution of methods and approaches is a practical response to the inductive nature of qualitative enquiry, which by its very nature is responsive to, and affected by, occurrences within the life of the study.

Concept summary: qualitative and quantitative differences

It is interesting to note at this point that both qualitative and quantitative researchers use quite similar data collection methods – such as interviews or observation. What differs between the two paradigms are what Sarantakos (2005) calls the 'methodological standards'. For the quantitative researcher, interviews follow a rigid and reproducible structure, with the same questions asked in the same way to a large number of people to gain quantifiable answers to a series of specific questions. For the qualitative researcher, each interview is unique, with intense questioning and a less formal structure. Questions might be open, and, depending on the answers from the respondents, new directions might be taken by the researcher.

Qualitative research methodologies have their roots in various associated academic disciplines and philosophical schools of thought. One of the common and enduring features of qualitative research is that the philosophies underpinning the methodological approach are evident in the design and execution of the study. When reading qualitative research studies it is not uncommon to see the researcher discuss the philosophical position they have adopted in the preamble to the study or at the very least state who or what has informed their approach.

Because of the human focus of both nursing and qualitative research, the focus of the NMC competency on practising autonomously and applying relevant research applies to qualitative research. In order to continue their development as competent professionals, nurses should familiarise themselves with the messages that qualitative research adds to the cumulative knowledge underpinning modern nursing practice.

The ESC that suggests nurses should be able to respond to their feedback from a wide range of sources, in order to learn, develop and improve 'services', reflects closely the messages learned from qualitative research. The issues that qualitative research often highlights are to do with the quality of the experience of care, so gaining an understanding of qualitative research methodologies links closely to the potential for improving nursing practice.

Concept summary: qualitative research

It is worth thinking for a moment about the philosophy underpinning qualitative research methodologies before exploring the questions they attempt to answer and the methods they employ. Qualitative research asks questions about the nature of reality; it regards reality as being both **subjective** and multiple. This means that qualitative researchers start from the viewpoint that reality is constructed by individuals from their interpretations of what is around them. This construction of reality is subject to personal interpretation and differs greatly from individual to individual. Indeed, the viewpoint of the individual can change over time and in response to life events – for example, becoming chronically ill.

A key characteristic of qualitative research that makes it different from quantitative research is that it does not try to **generalise** its findings (that is, it does not claim that because this is how one group of people see the world, then all people like them view the world in the same way). One way in which the researcher maintains a true reflection of the views and thoughts of the participants in the research is to represent what they have said word for word in the results, so that the meaning is not lost in interpretation.

The different qualitative methodologies have evolved to answer different questions. The questions that they answer are obviously related in some way to the academic disciplines from which they evolved (see Table 2.2). What this means for the qualitative researcher is not always clear and, as stated above, not all qualitative enquiry lends itself to being neatly pigeon-holed to one or other methodology. Often qualitative research is called just that – qualitative research – but the approach is normally informed by the assumptions of the paradigm or underpinning philosophy. This failure to identify an exact methodology is, in fact, not a failure at all. Rather, it is a response to the need to be flexible and pragmatic in order to achieve the aims of the study. The overarching philosophy, or more correctly **epistemology** (theory of knowledge), remains the same no matter which methodology is adopted (and even if no methodology at all is adopted). The nature of reality is both subjective and multiple.

The approach chosen to answer a qualitative question is at least in part dictated by the question itself. As can be seen in Table 2.3, there are some specific words associated with different research methodologies. For example, in phenomenology, the focus of which is on an in-depth understanding of a given phenomenon (or experience), the aim of the research is often stated as being to describe the essence of a phenomenon (essence in this sense can be thought of as similar

Table 2.2: The academic roots of the qualitative methodologies

Methodology	*Academic roots*
Ethnography	Sociology, cultural anthropology
Grounded theory	Sociology (specifically **symbolic interactionism**)
Phenomenology	Philosophy, psychology, sociology
Case study research	Social sciences

Table 2.3: Types of words used in the questions that different qualitative methodologies might be used to answer

Methodology	*Words used in questions*
Ethnography	Culture-sharing group, Behaviour, Language, Cultural portrait, Cultural themes.
Grounded theory	Generate, Develop, Propositions, Process, Substantive theory.
Phenomenology	Describe, Experiences, Meaning, Essence.
Case study research	Single or collective cases, Event, Process, Programme, Individual.

Source: adapted from Creswell (2007).

to the essence of a flavour used in cooking – for example, vanilla essence, which is the distilled down and essential flavour of vanilla). It is the understanding of the essence that points to, or from which might emerge, a greater understanding of the phenomenon of interest.

A further characteristic of qualitative research is that qualitative researchers try to get close to the person, or people, they are researching. The relationship between the researcher and the researched is part of the research process, and is fundamental to obtaining the insider perspective (**emic**) that qualitative research seeks. As well as getting close to the researched, the researcher also explores and expresses his or her own values about a topic of research before the research starts. This means that anyone reading the published research can form an opinion not only about what the researcher writes about the topic being investigated but also the reasons that they came to the conclusions they have.

Activity 2.2   *Reflection*

Try to remember what you thought it would be like to be a nurse before you came into the profession, and write down the ideas and preconceptions that you had. Now look at those ideas and preconceptions and see how they have changed and modified in relation to the experiences that you have had as a nurse. You will see that ideas and concepts change as a result of experience. Alternatively, ask a friend who is not a nurse to write down what they think nursing is all about and compare this to your current understanding.

An outline of what you might find is given at the end of the chapter.

Qualitative research is inductive in its approach to problem solving. 'Inductive' means that the research moves from a specific idea to something more general and theoretical (see Figure 1.2, page 13). The research question itself is quite broad and open. The inductive researcher does not set out with an idea of what they might find, as one does with a hypothesis, for example (see Figure 1.1 on page 12, and Chapter 4). Instead they allow the data they collect to lead them towards an understanding of the phenomenon under investigation. In grounded theory, for example, this inductive reasoning leads the researcher to the point where they create a new theory for understanding the social process under investigation.

Concept summary: inductive reasoning

If you are struggling with the concept of inductive reasoning, think about the methods employed by detectives in popular detective novels and television programmes (for example, Poirot or Miss Marple). These fictional detectives collect clues surrounding a given case and use these to construct hypotheses. At this stage they are acting inductively – they allow the information to lead them instead of looking for clues to support any preconceived notion about what might have happened. Once a number of clues have been gathered, the data are analysed and a hypothesis is formed; the detective then becomes more deductive, looking for clues and seeking out information that will support the hypothesis they have formed. This example not only demonstrates the differences between inductive and deductive approaches to research but it also demonstrates that the two can be used usefully together to help gain a full understanding of an individual or an occurrence.

Weaknesses of qualitative research

The very nature of qualitative research lays it open to many criticisms. The subjective nature of qualitative enquiry means that it is hard to replicate – that is to say, people's opinions and attitudes, beliefs and ideals are different from place to place and from time to time. So the opinions, attitudes, ideals and beliefs that are common in one setting are not necessarily the same in another because they are affected by nationality, culture and life experiences. Furthermore, subjectivity is so intertwined with context that a single event can change a person's perspective forever as the context of their life changes. This means that the findings of a qualitative study are inextricably linked to the people that were studied, the time in which they were studied and the prevalent cultural and social norms.

Activity 2.3   *Reflection*

What life events have changed your way of seeing the world? Life events are things that have happened to you or to others within your lifetime that affect your attitudes and opinions. Significant life events may include becoming a parent, experiencing illness or trauma or the death of a loved one. Other life events are experienced by people collectively and may include natural disasters or terrorist activity that change the way in which we see the world for ever.

How has your experience changed your view of things? Why?

An outline of what you might find is given at the end of the chapter.

The fact that the findings of qualitative research are so subjective and so bound to the context in which the research is undertaken means that the findings are hard to generalise. In turn, this means that it may be hard to justify applying the findings of any qualitative enquiry away from the setting in which the study was undertaken. That said, qualitative researchers claim, and rightly so, that the purpose of their enquiry is not necessarily to create findings that are statistically generalisable but to create what Popay et al. (1998) call *logical generalizations*, which relate to similar situations or occurrences. This means that the applicability of the findings of a qualitative study to a similar setting, or phenomenon, is not a matter of scientific certainty but a matter for careful thought and consideration within the relative context.

Qualitative research has also been criticised for lacking scientific **rigour** and credibility because the processes involved are subject to the values and beliefs of the person undertaking the research. Qualitative researchers counter this by saying that they recognise, and in some cases even welcome, the subjectivity of the qualitative research process. The fact that they acknowledge that their presence and actions within the research setting may affect the outcomes means that everyone is aware of the issue anyway, and that the results of the study can be read in this context. Or as Popay et al. state:

> *the question is not whether the data are biased, but to what extent has the researcher rendered transparent the processes by which data have been collected, analysed and presented.*
> (1998, p348)

Ethnography

Ethnographic research seeks to describe and interpret activity within social groups. It seeks to understand the culture within a group, where culture is defined as the behaviours, norms and meaning of the group from the viewpoint of an insider, that is, a member of the group (the emic perspective). Ethnography has its roots in **anthropology**, which literally means the study of humans and is taken from the Greek *anthropos* (human) and *logia* (study). Ethnography is used to study all manner of social relationships and realities, for example: understanding the impact of belief systems on the decision making of nurses working triage (Fry, 2012); considering the experiences of people managing their own diabetes (Hinder and Greenhalgh, 2012); gaining an insight into the construction of personal identity in society (Watson, 2012); and ascribing meaning to the experiences of newly qualified midwives as they develop their new identities (Hobbs, 2012).

Concept summary: emic perspective

An emic perspective is the insider's view. In ethnography this would be the view of the culture from a member of the group being studied. This is the opposite of the **etic** perspective, which is the view of someone else looking in at the same culture – in this case, perhaps, the ethnographer. If you are struggling with the concepts of emic and etic, think about how different people view political ideologies – for example, how a Labour party supporter would describe their party as opposed to how they might be described by a member of a different political group.

Key features

The key feature of ethnography as a qualitative research methodology is that it involves long-term study of a group by the researcher, who becomes both an observer and a participant in the group – this is often termed **participant observation**. Because the researchers are very much part of the group being studied, they will influence how the group behaves – and how the group behaves may influence them.

Tedlock (2001) observes that ethnographers may see their position as 'marginal natives' or 'professional strangers', or they may see themselves as 'going native' or 'maintaining some distance'. What this means is that ethnographers immerse themselves to different extents in the group being studied. Some maintain a professional and dispassionate distance (professional stranger) and try to maintain an air of objectivity. Other ethnographers become immersed in the culture they are studying and start not only to behave like the group being studied but to feel like and build emotional and social allegiances with the group (going native). Depending on your viewpoint, this 'going native' can be seen as either a problem or a benefit to the research process.

Case study

James Patrick, who studied gang culture in Glasgow in the 1950s, left Glasgow in a hurry after only 12 sessions with the gang from the Maryhill district of the city. Patrick had found the level of violence unacceptable and was unable to study the gang any longer. He did, however, manage to publish his study of the gang's culture after a suitable period of time, which served to protect the gang members' identities (Patrick, 1973).

Sampling in ethnographic research

Access to a group for study may involve the researcher in seeking the help of a **gatekeeper**. In this sense, a gatekeeper is someone already in a group who will not only allow them access to the group but also introduce them to group members and even help them to integrate into the group. Classically, researchers have downplayed their own role in a group in an attempt to maintain some level of objectivity, or artificial distance, and **credibility**. However, it is now more common for researchers to explore their own part in the group as part of the research – in a sense creating their own autobiography of belonging to the group.

Some ethnographers use their place of work as a rich source of data for ethnography, seeking to derive meaning from the interactions that take place there. In this context, the ability and opportunities for data collection are vast and the insights gained may be great. There are some issues with this approach, however, as one may start off 'native' and therefore lack objectivity and there remain ethical questions about the informed consent of colleagues who may forget that they are now subject to study as well as being colleagues in the classic sense.

Case study

In her case study seeking to understand the meaning newly qualified midwives placed on their experiences in the workplace, Hobbs (2012) undertook a participant observation of seven newly qualified staff (a ***purposive*** *sample). She maintained a reflexive field diary of her observations and interviews undertaken in the workplace. Her observations and interviews allowed her to gain an insight into the professional and cultural experiences of the participants within their new working environments. This allows for changes to be made in the induction and training of new midwives in order to improve their experience of the transition from student to midwife as well as their ability to provide good-quality patient care.*

Methods used in data collection

Data collection in ethnography focuses on three key activities: what the people in the group are doing; the things that have meaning to the group and what those things are; and what the people in the group say (Spradley, 1980). In order to collect these data the ethnographer therefore engages with the group in a number of different ways.

Activity 2.4   *Critical thinking*

Given that ethnographers are often studying groups about which they have little knowledge, and with whom they have few connections, what problems might they encounter when trying to collect data for their study? How might they overcome some of these problems? Do you think it is possible to remain entirely objective at the same time as immersing oneself in the activities of the group being studied?

There is a possible answer at the end of the chapter.

Participant observation is the key method used in data collection. Being part of a group allows the researcher to gain a perspective on the norms of the group, its use of language and its shared values. The ethnographer keeps copious notes of the interactions within the group and between themselves and members of the group, often reflecting on and deciphering meaning from seemingly casual conversations and interactions. Gathering and reflecting on information requires a level of practised detachment on the part of the researcher that allows them to see meaning within normal everyday interactions.

It would be reasonable to ask at this point what the purpose of prolonged observation is. Surely any insights can be gained during interviews or focus group discussions? Verbal data-collection methods have an important role to play in the understanding of the group. There are, however, things that groups may share a common knowledge or understanding of that they may not think important and would therefore not raise during interview. Such things, often termed **tacit knowledge**, may not be raised in conversation but will emerge from the interactions of the group. One of the important roles of ethnography is to discover, and describe, this sort of important hidden detail.

Concept summary: tactit knowledge

Tacit knowledge is a common feature of nursing (and, indeed, many professions). There are understandings that we gain about human interaction and the delivery of care that we know, but just don't know why we know them. Not only do we forget why we may know something but we also sometimes forget where we learnt it. As such, this knowledge is then just part of our body of knowledge as nurses – something that does not usually need to be discussed within our professional body but that is unknown to others outside nursing. It might be described as knowing as a result of informal social learning. A word of caution, however: tacit knowledge could be inaccurate if the initial set of actions is wrong and this learning goes unchallenged, for example where new knowledge is not subjected to critical reflection.

Other data collected may include pictures, symbols and images that have meaning to the members of the group and that allow the researcher to convey these meanings to the people reading their research. Such symbols may give clues to the shared understandings and identity of the group and promote deeper understanding.

More structured data collection is a common feature of ethnographic studies, which often means undertaking interviews. Because of the long-term relationships developed during the course of a study, interviews may actually occur during everyday conversations and interactions. Many ethnographers use in-depth formal interviews during the course of their data collection, employing **open questions** that are designed to allow the respondent to answer in whatever way they feel is correct without leading them towards an answer.

It is easy to imagine from this description that data collection proceeds in a well-defined and planned manner; however, this certainly is not always the case. Indeed, the three key activities of data collection described above happen simultaneously and cyclically. As such, data collection in ethnography can be quite messy and challenging, and requires detailed note taking, constant reflection, and development and amendment of methods depending on what is found, when and how.

Grounded theory

Grounded theory is a qualitative methodology that is used to analyse social processes that occur within human interactions. It can be thought of as a methodology that tries to generate new, or explore and expand upon existing ideas or 'theories' about a human activity by examining people's perceptions and understandings of social interactions. Once the theory is derived, its application to a social interaction can be viewed as providing a potential explanation of the important social processes that have been derived (grounded) from the data collected.

Grounded theory research is used to generate theories about practice and understanding from many different areas of healthcare, including: generating an understanding of the experiences of the onset of anorexia in young people (Koruth et al., 2012); creating an understanding of the role identity of health visitors in the UK in the light of the changes to their changing practice context (Machin et al., 2012); and exploring the experiences and views about end-of-life care of people affected with terminal lung cancer and their family members (Horne et al., 2012).

Key features

Of the qualitative approaches to research, grounded theory is perhaps the most systematic in its approach. Philosophically and academically it is closely linked to sociology, the study of people in society and social groups. Grounded theory is one of the most popular qualitative methodologies used by nurse researchers.

The whole grounded theory approach to enquiry is based on the notion that a social group, or groups, have shared social interpretations that are not always well described (Glaser and Strauss, 1967). Barney Glaser and Anselm Strauss, the founders of modern grounded theory, expressly criticised sociology because at the time sociologists were seeking evidence to support existing theories rather than using evidence to create new theory. Glaser and Strauss's argument, quite reasonably, suggested that if sociology was to accept that a theory had any basis in truth, then the data for the generation of the theory, which in social and natural science means something more than a hunch or speculation, had to precede the creation of the theory and not the other way round! In this way the philosophy underpinning grounded theory is very inductive.

Grounded theory systematically applies procedural steps to explore social phenomena and derive a theory that explains people's understanding of those phenomena. Strauss and Corbin (1990, p23) explain a grounded theory as:

> *one that is inductively derived from the study of the phenomenon it represents. That is, it is discovered, developed, and provisionally verified through systematic data collection and analysis of data pertaining to that phenomenon. Therefore, data collection, analysis, and theory stand in reciprocal relationship with each other. One does not begin with a theory, then prove it. Rather, one begins with an area of study and what is relevant to that area is allowed to emerge.*

The aim of grounded theory is, therefore, the discovery of theoretical explanations for and about a particular phenomenon.

Concept summary: inductive and deductive reasoning

Individuals who use inductive reasoning believe that concepts, theories and ideas are created from empirical (sensory) observations. They work from what they observe, and the data they collect, to the idea. This is the opposite to deductive reasoning, which involves collecting data to prove a hypothesis or idea. Francis Bacon, one of the great philosophers of the seventeenth century, claimed that the important knowledge we have as humans derives from inductive methods taking as their starting point empirical observation.

Like ethnography, then, grounded theory focuses on meanings coming out from the phenomena being studied, rather than on forming a hypothesis before starting the study. Grounded theory, however, is regarded more as a theory-building strategy in social science research. Ethnographers usually do not interpret or derive meaning from their observations and interviews but allow them to stand unchallenged, whereas grounded theorists will look for evidence to support, or refute, the theory being built.

Concept summary: theories and hypotheses

At this point it is worth thinking about the nature of a **theory** and a **hypothesis**. The word hypothesis can be thought of as a combination of the two words 'hypo' (below) and 'thesis' (well-developed idea), while a theory may be regarded as a hypothesis that is supported by the collection of evidence such that it is closer to being established fact. It is important when thinking about the nature of qualitative enquiry using the grounded theory methodology that the ultimate aim is to generate a theory, that is, an idea or concept supported by empirical facts.

Sampling in grounded theory research

A **homogeneous** sample of people who have all shared the same experience, or gone through the same process, is the starting point for sampling for grounded theory research. The sample is, therefore, purposive (selected for the purpose of the study). The sample needs to be broad enough to enable the researcher to draw on the experiences of enough people to come to some conclusions about the commonalities of the experience. Often a **convenience sample** will be used, which consists of people who are identified because they attend a particular hospital clinic, social group or perhaps a university course.

After interviewing the initial sample the grounded theorist will analyse the interviews for the data that emerge and start to create initial theories about the phenomenon of interest (for more about this process in grounded theory, see Chapter 3). This initial and ongoing analysis of data will lead researchers to ask further questions around the area of interest and may lead to them recruiting further subjects to the study in order to help answer emerging questions or to further consolidate an emerging theory. This process is called **theoretical sampling**.

Concept summary: theoretical sampling

Theoretical sampling is a sampling method that is usually confined to grounded theory research. Theoretical sampling occurs as researchers build new theories and ideas from the data they have collected; they test these new theories by interviewing more subjects to see if the new theories still hold true. Theoretical sampling is also known as 'handy' sampling.

Methods used in data collection

Grounded theorists collect data from a variety of sources, including case studies, interviews, documentary evidence and participant observation. Interviews remain the most widely used mechanism of data collection because it is only during interview that the researcher can get to the heart of the individual's interpretation of a phenomenon. In order to get to such meaning the interviews are usually in-depth and **unstructured** or **semi-structured**, to allow the interviewer to respond to the ideas and statements coming from the participant rather than boxing the interviewee in by the use of questions that may be irrelevant to the individual.

Case study

The grounded theory research by Horne et al. (2012) sought to explore the priorities people with terminal illness have about end-of-life care and how these shape their views on the end of life itself. The study included 25 terminally ill patients and 19 of their family members and identified, through semi-structured interviews, that people prioritise the social aspects of their death over and above the medical and that they had a strong desire to live in the here and now.

Grounded theory research methods are well structured and well developed, and it is hard to separate the process of data collection from the process of data analysis since what one finds determines to a large extent for how long one continues to collect data. Data collection and analysis take place simultaneously. This process informs the sampling that continues until no new data to inform the emergent (grounded) theory is forthcoming.

Phenomenology

Phenomenology has a short, colourful and somewhat eclectic history. Phenomenology has variously been applied to the study of people, ethics, law, aesthetics and architecture (Moran, 2000). There are a number of distinct philosophical tendencies within phenomenology, but at their heart lies the definition of phenomenology as: *The study of structures of consciousness as experienced from the first person point of view* (Smith, 2004).

It is this requisite of accessing the nature of the 'first person' experience that lies at the heart of phenomenology, which establishes its strong emic credentials. In health and social care phenomenology is widely used to aid understanding of such phenomena as giving birth when the mother has a spinal cord injury (Tebbet and Kennedy, 2012); understanding the personal meaning residents of care homes give to the fact that the people they live with regularly die (Djivre et al., 2012); and exploring the dietary choices among people who have survived a myocardial infarction (Doyle et al., 2012)

Key features

Edmund Husserl is credited as being the founder of modern phenomenology; his method of studying human consciousness and experience is characterised by an approach that is often termed **descriptive phenomenology**. Husserl's approach relied heavily on the fact that humans are by nature reflective beings who make sense of their world using the evidence available to them via their physical senses. The purpose of descriptive phenomenology is to access the essence of an object or an experience as the individual experiencing it sees it – no more and no less – what Crotty (1998) describes as the ultimate structure of consciousness. While accessing this experience through the research subject (usually via interview), the researcher puts out of their mind any preconceived ideas they have about the object or experience, a process known as **epoching** or **bracketing** (Zahavi, 2003).

Of course, in reality it is virtually impossible to put to one side one's feelings or one's prior knowledge of an event or an experience, and most phenomenological researchers actually describe their own preconceptions about an issue being researched prior to starting the data collection. This 'laying bare', as it is called, allows anyone else reading the research to judge for themselves whether the preconceived ideas of the researcher have had an impact on their interpretation of what the research subjects have said.

> **Concept summary: epoching**
>
> Epoching or bracketing is the process by which the researcher puts to one side all of their preconceptions and ideas about the topic they are studying. By putting aside all pre-conceived ideas about the world or the phenomenon being studied, the researcher can allow the inductive process of coming to an understanding of things through the use of the data as they emerge to take place. Some commentators liken this to putting your ideas and preconceptions into your pocket.

Martin Heidegger, a student of Husserl's, modified the descriptive phenomenological approach. His **interpretative phenomenology** is refined by his attention to the **hermeneutics**, or analysis/interpretation, of human experience. Unlike Husserl's approach, Heidegger's view is that human existence, and experience, is made up of our interpretations of what we see, feel and experience (Parahoo, 2006). Hence, Heidegger's hermeneutical phenomenology relies heavily on accessing the individual's expressed perspective on their lived experience, which is intertwined with and influenced by their social context. Heidegger believed our understanding comes from *being-in-the-world*, a key to understanding the experiences of others (Dreyfus, 1991).

More recently, **interpretative phenomenological analysis** (IPA) has attempted to work with, rather than round, the interpretative nature of phenomenological enquiry. The emphasis remains on accessing the participants' perception of the phenomenon, but it further recognises that this is itself an interpretation of the lived world and that the researcher will themselves apply an interpretation to the research subjects' interpretation (Smith and Osborn, 2004). That is, the researcher will try to make sense of the subjects' attempts to make sense of their world.

Streubert Speziale and Carpenter (2007) helpfully identify three questions that the researcher should ask before setting out to undertake a phenomenological study. First, is there a need for more clarity of understanding of the phenomenon? Second, will the experiences of the subjects provide this information? Third, have I got the time, resources, skills and personality necessary to undertake this study?

The first and second questions help in deciding if the approach is the right one; they eliminate doubt about the need for and the approach to answering the question posed. The third question is more practical and could apply equally well to any research enquiry (as discussed at the end of Chapter 1). The nature of phenomenology, however, is such that it requires the researcher to engage with the process in a great deal of depth, over a long period of time, while recognising their own biases and personal opinions.

Sampling in phenomenological research

The sampling method used in phenomenological research has, by definition, to be a **purposive** one. Purposive samples select people who have experienced the phenomenon of interest. So, for example, if one wanted to know what it was like to have multiple sclerosis, then one would approach and research people who have the disease. The sample selection will be determined by the exact question that one is seeking to answer. So, again, if one were interested in what it was like to be a mother living with multiple sclerosis, then one would approach only mothers who were living with the disease.

In common with all qualitative methodologies, phenomenology seeks to gain in-depth understanding of a topic that is credible and might extrapolate to similar situations. **Generalisability** (the ability to generalise the findings of a study beyond the sample researched) is not as important in qualitative research as it is in quantitative, and therefore, as in all qualitative methods, the samples used are generally quite small. Various sources suggest that a sample of between 6 and 20 individuals is sufficient for the purposes of this kind of study (Polkinghorne, 1989). In reality, the sample size may be determined by time, money and availability of study subjects. As with many qualitative studies, a convenience sample is often used. Also in common with other qualitative study samples, because of the in-depth nature of this type of study the small sample can provide data that are both rich and deep, reflecting the intended purpose of qualitative methodologies.

Perhaps the ideal way to determine the size of the sample to be studied in phenomenological research is to analyse the data from the interviews as the study progresses, stopping the interview process when no new themes are emerging from the data. The point at which there appears to be no new ideas emerging from the interviews is often referred to as **data saturation**.

Concept summary: data saturation

Data saturation is a term used in many qualitative methodologies to define the point at which there appears to be no further benefit to be gained from continuing to collect data about a topic of interest. The use of data saturation as identifying the point at which data collection stops is as much practical as academic. This is because qualitative methodologies (unlike quantitative methodologies) cannot use statistical sample size calculations as a point at which to stop the collection of data for a study because they are not concerned with collecting numerate data.

Methods used in data collection

Data for phenomenological research are almost invariably collected using interviews. The reason for this is that interviews allow the researcher to explore in depth an issue with an individual by adjusting their questioning according to what the respondent is saying, probing the meaning behind the responses given and thereby gaining insight into the experience of the individual.

Case study

In their phenomenological study of seeking to understand why so many people who survive a myocardial infarction (heart attack) do not alter their eating behaviours, Doyle et al. (2012) interviewed nine attendees from a post-myocardial infarction rehabilitation clinic. They uncovered some enabling themes around fear of recurrence, determination and self-control that drove dietary changes, while poor recall, the need for more support and lack of willpower prevented some participants from changing their eating behaviours.

Phenomenological studies often use either unstructured or semi-structured interview methodologies (as opposed to the more rigid structured interview that might be undertaken as part of market research). More flexible interviewing structures allow the interview to explore the issues that are of importance to the interviewee. This exploratory interview method fits better with the aims of phenomenological research, which are to explore the meaning or essence of an experience (such as the reasons for dietary choices made following a myocardial infarction) for the individual. Open questions are used (also called open-ended questions).

Some researchers have used focus groups as a means of collecting data for phenomenological studies. While these are quicker than a series of one-to-one interviews, the disadvantage is that they collect a group consensus view and may not always gain insight into the actual feelings or interpretations of the individuals present. These difficulties may be more acute when the topic being researched is in a sensitive area.

Case study/biographic research

Creswell (2007, p73) defines case study research as: *an exploration of a 'bounded system' or a case (or multiple cases) over time through detailed, in-depth data collection involving multiple sources of information rich in context.* While this definition is correct, it may appear to be misleading since Creswell is using the term 'bounded system' to refer to any of the following: an individual, a collection of individuals, a system, an organisation or an intervention.

Case study research is perhaps the least well understood approach to qualitative enquiry. It is a widely held view among the research community that case study research is not useful as an insight into a wider group or other systems and that its usefulness is restricted to the early stage of qualitative enquiry in hypothesis generation to be tested by subsequent larger-scale investigations. In their qualitative case study McNeil et al. (2012) explored the nature of end-of-life care for homeless and marginalised individuals; Lorentzen et al. (2012) identified some of the reactions and attitudes of overweight children and their families grappling to change their diets; while Meffe et al. (2012) studied the impact of an interprofessional maternity care education programme on the knowledge, skills and attitudes of participants.

Key features

According to Yin (2008), a case study approach to qualitative questioning might be considered when: the point of the study is answering 'how' and 'why' questions; it is not possible to manipulate the behaviour of the individuals involved in the study; the boundaries between the phenomenon and context are unclear; it is desirable to study the contextual conditions because it is believed that they are of relevance to the phenomenon being studied.

Sampling in case study research

In common with most qualitative methods, the starting point for the sample for the research are individuals who constitute the system being researched or have experience of the intervention of interest that is purposive. Some research commentators, Cresswell (2007) among them, consider that sampling unusual cases (those whose experience of the topic under discussion is not the norm) is useful in some collective case studies as they provide a broader perspective on the issue. What is clear in case study research is that a lot of thought needs to go into what exactly one is studying because there is a world of difference between studying an individual and studying a process or organisation.

Methods used in data collection

A feature of case study research is the use of multiple sources of data. Potential sources of data include documentation, interviews, archived records, objects, observation and pictures. Unlike other qualitative research methodologies, case study researchers can use quantitative data in order to gain a fuller insight into a phenomenon being studied. Data from the many different sources are then joined together in the analysis, rather like putting together the pieces of a puzzle.

Bringing the pieces of the puzzle together like this allows the researcher to gain a more holistic view of the individual or system being studied. Bringing together data from many different sources adds strength to the findings as the various strands of enquiry are woven together to improve upon the understanding of the phenomenon under study.

Of course, there is always the potential pitfall with this type of eclectic approach that too much data will be collected and that it will prove too overwhelming to process all the data in a meaningful manner. To this end there are many advantages of using a computerised database for case study research.

Case study

In their case study research into the impact of interprofessional education for maternity care, Meffe et al. (2012) used repeated interviews with nine participants over a 20-month period. They demonstrated that educating nurses, midwives and medical students together appeared to have positive benefits in terms of the relationships between the professions, their interprofessional communication, their willingness to work in a collaborative manner and their women-centredness.

In their case study of the culture of an intensive care unit, Storesund and McMurray (2009) used semi-structured interviews to gain their insight into the culture of an intensive care unit. The study showed the nurses to have identified three key influences on the quality of nursing: preserving cohesiveness despite the complicated and stressful nature of the job; quick, focused and respectful communication; and having expert knowledge, achieved through both clinical experience and formal learning.

Chapter summary

In this chapter we have seen that qualitative research usually has at its heart the creation of knowledge in an inductive fashion. This knowledge focuses on understanding human experience using a variety of methods that involve getting close to, and understanding, the way in which various people experience and make sense of their worlds.

We have identified the major methodologies that are used within qualitative research in healthcare and have discovered that not all qualitative research is clearly based on one specific methodology. We have seen that qualitative research is used to answer a number of different questions, and certain methodologies and methods are best suited to specific types of question. The ways in which samples are chosen – and the reasons for these – have been identified, as have the key methods used to collect data in qualitative research.

We have seen that qualitative research is important to nursing in extending our understanding of how people experience the care that we deliver. If we review the key messages of qualitative research, it is straightforward to see how an understanding of the approaches to and tools used in qualitative research add an additional dimension to our ability as nurses to deliver high-quality care.

Activities: Brief outline answers

Activity 2.2: Reflection (page 28)

It is likely that your perceptions of nursing have changed as you have gained experience in the practice setting. Alternatively, you should be able to see a difference between how you see the activity of nursing and the perceptions of someone who is not themselves a nurse. Undoubtedly, experience of something changes our perceptions of it as the realities of the experience create more concrete understanding on which to base our insights.

Activity 2.3: Reflection (page 29)

Life experiences all have an effect on the person that we become. While nurses are often encouraged to be empathetic towards their patients it is hard to become so without some life experiences to draw on. Experiencing life-changing events such as pain, embarrassment or bereavement allow us to better understand what some of our patients experience while they are in our care.

Activity 2.4: Critical thinking (page 32)

Getting into, and understanding the values, of a group requires the ethnographer to establish a rapport with a member of the group of interest (a gatekeeper). This group member then becomes their means of gaining access to the group and may help the researcher to identify the shared values and common understandings of the group. This is not always easy as many groups have a language of their own and share a common understanding of issues, symbols and ideas not immediately obvious to an outsider. Think about the language you are used to in the practice setting and how hard it was to sit through a handover when you were new to nursing. The key to success is, therefore, time and communication with a key informant within the group who can give meaning to new ideas, processes and concepts in much the same way as a clinical mentor does for the student nurse. The ability to remain objective during data collection for an ethnographic study will be affected by the amount of time and the intensity of the new experience. For the novice researcher this may be achieved by using a research supervisor or a research buddy who can provide a sounding board and a reality check when needed.

Further reading

Creswell, JW (2007) *Qualitative inquiry and research design: choosing among five approaches*. Thousand Oaks CA: Sage.

A great text for understanding the differences between the qualitative research methodologies.

Parahoo, K (2006) *Nursing research: principles, process and issues* (2nd edn). London: Palgrave Macmillan.

Chapter 4 is a very useful introduction to the principles of qualitative research.

Streubert Speziale, HJ and Carpenter, DR (2007) *Qualitative research in nursing: advancing the humanistic imperative* (4th edn). London: Lippincott Williams & Wilkins.

Chapters 1 and 2 provide a very accessible introduction to the philosophy and conduct of qualitative research.

Useful websites

www.analytictech.com/mb870/introtoGT.htm An introduction to grounded theory.

www.phenomenologycenter.org An easy-to-use site regarding phenomenological research, from the Center for Advanced Research in Phenomenology.

www.qualres.org/ A comprehensive website covering all aspects of qualitative research.

www.statisticalassociates.com/groundedtheory.pdf A nice, and free, guide to grounded theory as a downloadable book.

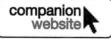

For further activities and other useful material, visit the companion website at **www.sagepub.co.uk/ellis_research2e**

Chapter 3
Data collection methods and analysis in qualitative research

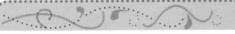
Chapter aims

After reading this chapter, you will be able to:

*   identify the major data collection methods employed in qualitative research;
*   describe the advantages and disadvantages of the data collection methods used in qualitative research;

- describe the key elements of data analysis in qualitative research;
- demonstrate awareness of the quality issues related to data management in qualitative research.

Introduction

In the previous chapter qualitative research methodologies were identified as a means of answering questions about people's opinions, attitudes, feelings and interpretation of experience. This chapter identifies the appropriate data collection methods within qualitative research and explains how they meet the aims of the chosen methodology. It will explore how the data are collected, and the pros and cons of the verbal and observational data collection methods within the qualitative methodologies.

The aim of this chapter is to introduce the reader to the general principles of the approaches and some of their strengths and weaknesses rather than to provide an exhaustive exploration of the methods used in qualitative research. Readers are advised to access the further reading suggested at the end of the chapter if they want further information or guidance on the application of qualitative research methods.

This chapter also looks at data presentation and data analysis in qualitative research and what they serve to demonstrate. It also illuminates some of the ways in which the process of data analysis in the qualitative methodologies can be demonstrated to be **rigorous** and **credible**, that is to say, how the quality of the data collection is demonstrated.

Key features

It is clear that the qualitative methodologies are concerned with people, the actions of people and the meaning that people attach to the activities in which they engage. Capturing people's behaviour and the meanings they attach to it is not something that can be undertaken lightly or superficially. Qualitative researchers often argue that the work that they do is both deep and rich.

This depth and richness, which is sometimes referred to as 'thickness' (Streubert Speziale and Carpenter, 2007), comes from the ability of the methodologies and their associated methods to tap into the meaning of human interaction and of being. These notions are not readily measurable in an empirical sense, nor can they be identified by casual observation or interaction.

Clearly, any attempt to understand human interaction – or people's understanding of, or feelings about a topic – requires engagement with the individuals in question. This allows the researcher to gain an insight into the world of the research participant and the meaning they attach to the things that happen there. Engaging with, and understanding, people takes time, effort and some perseverance.

As nurses, we are familiar and comfortable with the day-to-day communications and interactions that take place between us and our patients. We undertake clinical observations and gather data to inform our care. The interaction required for qualitative data collection is somewhat deeper than that required in the general nursing setting. Such interactions require not only observation and our interpretation of the observation, but also probing and understanding of the topic from the point of view of the subject of the research.

Concept summary: signs and symptoms

In order to think about the difference between your understanding of the world and someone else's understanding of the world, think about the difference between signs and symptoms of illness. Signs are things that we can measure and see in other people, for instance their temperature, pulse and blood pressure. Symptoms have to be explained to us by the person experiencing them, for example pain or anxiety. So to gain an insight into someone else's world, we need to ask them how they see things, what their experience is and how they interpret it. We cannot gain this just by looking at them, in the same way that we cannot see the symptoms of their illness!

The collection of data within the qualitative methods therefore requires in-depth engagement on the part of the researcher. The researcher is seen as a 'tool of data collection' rather than as someone who uses tools to collect data (as one might use a thermometer when taking a temperature or a sphygmomanometer for recording blood pressure, for example). This is seen as both a key strength and a key weakness of data collection in qualitative research.

The main strength lies in the depth of the data that can be collected, and the main weakness is that it is hard to either prevent or detect bias in the data collection. The quality of the processes by which bias is controlled in qualitative data collection and analysis is referred to as its rigour (Macnee and McCabe, 2008).

Concept summary: rigour

Rigour refers to the strict processes attached to both data collection and analysis within qualitative research that establishes their credibility and the dependability of the findings. The consistency and quality of the data collection processes, the manner in which these are recorded and described, and the quality of the data analysis, as well as its transparency, all add to the rigour that a study can be said to have. A good study will demonstrate that it has been thoroughly rigorous; a poor study will leave questions about the level of rigour used.

The next section of the chapter explores verbal data collection methods, i.e. interviews and focus groups. After that, observation – primarily participant observation – as a tool of qualitative data is discussed.

Interviews

There are a number of ways in which interviews can be undertaken in qualitative research. The choice of interview method, number of interviews and place of interview will depend on the nature of the issue being examined and the experience of the researcher. It would be misleading to state that a particular style of interviewing belongs to a specific qualitative methodology, as there is limited agreement on this issue even among experienced researchers – although, as we will see, the questions posed by some qualitative methodologies do tend to suggest that one approach to interviewing is used in preference to another.

Interviewing for qualitative research is a skill that requires acquisition and development as it improves with practice. Before undertaking an interview there are a number of questions the interviewer needs to ask and answer. Not least among these is 'What is the purpose of the interview?' This may seem a simplistic question at first glance, but it is one with clear links to the question posed in the study and the choice of research methodology.

In one form of phenomenological research, for example, the interviewer will be seeking to gain a deep insight into the 'essence' of the experience being investigated. The nature of the enquiry and the in-depth understanding required would tend to suggest that the interview (or interviews) needs to be lengthy and probing. By way of contrast, the conversations and data collection the ethnographer undertakes may range from informal or casual conversations to more structured and probing in-depth interviews, depending on the original question.

Despite specific methods apparently belonging to specific methodologies, different researchers will choose to use different data collection methods to answer their research questions even when apparently working within the same methodology. We have already seen that in-depth interviews are widely used in phenomenological research; however, Bradbury-Jones et al. (2009) argue that the use of focus groups in phenomenological research can be beneficial as it opens up the participants to alternative views while stimulating discussion about the topic of interest. Being subjected to other views and opinions can, they claim, improve understanding and hence refine the views of the participants, leading to higher-quality data collection. Conversely, it may be argued that this potential changing of the opinions and understanding of the participants is contrary to the purpose of phenomenological study, which is to see the world as others see it.

Interviews are appropriate when the research question seeks to discover the thoughts, feelings or perceptions of individuals about an issue or experience. They can be used to add context to other data collected during a study by adding an element of interpretation to something observed, for example, in an ethnographic enquiry. They are also beneficial when the topic being investigated is one that may cause embarrassment or that people are likely to be reserved about discussing in a group setting (Tod, 2006).

> ## Activity 3.1   *Reflection*
>
> Think about how easy it is to discuss sensitive issues in the open ward. How do you approach making it easier for patients to tell you private and intimate details in the practice setting? What barriers exist to gaining a full and frank insight into the thoughts and feelings of the patients where you work?
>
> *There are some possible answers at the end of the chapter.*

Key features

Interviewing as a data collection method requires prior planning. By the time the researcher has got to the point of planning the interview they should already have identified the purpose of the interview and the sample characteristics needed, and have some rough idea of the sample size.

Planning the interview requires the researcher to be clear about what information is wanted and from whom. This relates back strongly to the purpose of the study and the study question, which should guide the whole research process. The people being interviewed, and the nature of the research, will guide the nature of the interviewing process. For example, research with children may require the interview to be short and well structured. When interviewing adults, the process might benefit from allowing more time and being less structured in its approach to allow the interviewees' ideas and thoughts to be fully expressed and explored.

The philosophical basis of the study and the nature of the question to be asked will have the greatest bearing on the choice of interview type. Interviews may vary from short structured surveys with precise, often **closed questions** (as you might find in a survey) through to unstructured and **open questions** that are primarily exploratory (as in phenomenology or grounded theory).

> **Concept summary: open and closed questions**
>
> Open questions are questions that do not suggest any sort of answer. They are a good way of starting a long and involved conversation. Open questions may start with phrases such as 'tell me about. . .' or 'describe to me. . .'. They focus on the what, why and how of human experience and understanding. They allow the respondent to take the lead in setting the direction in which the interview will go.
>
> Closed questions are questions that suggest an answer or answers and invite only a limited range of responses. These may be 'yes', 'no' or factual answers such as one's age or town of residence. Closed questions may feature in later stages of a piece of research, and be used as a way of exploring the amount of agreement with an idea or theory a researcher has formed from earlier open questioning.

Interviews usually take place in a private setting. The exact location depends on the nature of the interviews, the people being interviewed and other practical considerations. Often the interviews will take place in a room at a university or hospital, although for some purposes the home of the interviewee may be more appropriate.

Qualitative interviews can last anything from half an hour up to about an hour and a half, although some may take much longer. If an interview is any shorter than this, it will fail to achieve satisfactory depth. Longer interviews risk tiring both the interviewer and the interviewee, making them more likely to wander from the point. Again, the nature of the research, the interviewees and the questions that are being answered by the research determine the length of the interview, as will issues such as the availability of the researcher and the interviewee.

In qualitative research, interviews usually require the interviewer to become close to the interviewee and to engage with what they are saying, rather than trying to control the interview (Sarantakos, 2005). This is in direct contrast to data collection methods used in quantitative research where researchers must keep themselves as distant as possible from the research subjects while maintaining control over all aspects of the research process.

That said, while the interview needs to be 'open', it will require some direction in order that the time the interviewer has with the interviewee is used to its maximum potential. Indeed, Parahoo (2006) points out that in reality no interview can be entirely unstructured. This is logical since the interview has a purpose that will in some way guide the conversation to be about the issue being explored.

All interviews should be recorded wherever possible, although a casual conversation in ethnography, for example, may not lend itself to this. The recording of the interview is generally important as it allows the researcher to capture word for word – **verbatim** – what the interviewee is saying. This means that there is no chance of the researcher forgetting something that has been said. Recording the interview also frees the researcher from having to take copious notes during the process, allowing them to concentrate on the content of the interview itself (Whiting, 2008). The recording is then transcribed (that is, typed up) – again verbatim – to allow the researcher to read through the resulting transcript many times in order to identify the important issues raised.

It is crucial to establish the ground rules associated with an interview. These rules will cover anonymity and confidentiality. It is important to establish that the anonymity of the interviewee will be preserved throughout the research process, subject to the disclosures being legal and depending on local data protection rules. This will usually mean that the transcripts of the interview are given a code to identify the interviewee rather than being labelled with their name.

In health and social care, where issues of harm, potential harm or illegal behaviour are identified in an interview, it may be necessary to disclose these to someone in authority. The interviewee should understand this before the interview takes place. It is never acceptable for a nurse researcher to ignore legal or ethical issues that would cause concern in their day-to-day nursing practice just because they are engaged in research. For example, the disclosure of the abuse of a child or vulnerable adult or the threat of violence towards another person would require that the researcher brought the issue to the attention of the relevant authorities.

As well as recording the interview, it is also important to write notes about the setting of the interview, the interviewee's body language and other non-verbal communications. Since the majority of human communication is non-verbal (Burgoon et al., 1996), these notes are an important tool in capturing the true meaning of the interview, and they provide context for the later analysis.

Activity 3.2   *Research and finding out*

When you are next in the clinical setting, spend some time silently observing the interactions between staff and patients, visitors and patients, staff and staff. Without listening in to the conversations, what can you tell about them from your observations? How can you tell that a patient is in pain or anxious without asking? What does this tell you about the nature of human communication?

There are some possible answers at the end of the chapter.

In some cases it is appropriate to video record the interview to allow for the later analysis of the interaction – including all of the non-verbal communication. Despite the ready availability of video recording technology, the video recording of interviews remains unusual, with many researchers believing that it serves to put the interviewee less at ease than the more usual voice recording method.

There are also ethical and practical issues associated with video recording that have to be taken into account. For example, it is difficult to exclude other people from a video if it is made in a public place, and some people will feel more vulnerable when filmed than when voice recorded even if the filming is done in private. Again, the nature of the research question, the people being interviewed and practical considerations have to drive the decision about how any interview will be recorded.

Advantages

The key advantage of interviews is that they allow the exploration of a topic in more depth and have the potential to create rich data. This is certainly true when they are compared to surveys and questionnaires, for example. Interviews allow the interviewer to respond to and probe the responses that a participant has given and also to tailor the interview to what they hear (Sarantakos, 2005).

As interviews are usually face to face, they allow the interviewer to both respond to and collect data about participants' body language during the questioning process. These data are helpful in establishing whether the interview subjects are happy to talk about the subject under investigation, and whether they appear to be answering in a truthful way, seem to be hiding something or are answering in a manner that they think the interviewer wants to hear (Tod, 2006).

Interviews allow the interviewer to explain the meaning of a question or to rephrase it in a way that the interviewee understands if this is needed. This is a real strength over a self-completion questionnaire where the respondent either may not understand a question or may feel that the options available for answering do not represent their feelings or thoughts. Being able to explain a question also means that interviews can be used as a means of data collection where the interviewees have limited literacy skills (Tod, 2006).

Interviews are a very human process; they mimic day-to-day conversation, and in doing so they can be made to feel comfortable for the interviewee, making them more likely to answer the questions they are asked. A skilled interviewer uses all the talents of a practised nurse in communicating with the interviewee, establishing a rapport and putting the interviewee at ease (something that it is hard to do when not face to face).

Disadvantages

All of the disadvantages of interviews can be avoided by careful preparation and management of the process. The lack of prior experience of interviewing is perhaps a major drawback. Although it is hard to get real life experience of observing an interview, the novice researcher can read and listen to examples of interviews and learn some of the strategies in this way. The use of a topic guide or list of questions to be covered in the interview can help novice interviewers to achieve what they need from the interview process.

Interviews can be prone to a form of bias, where the person being interviewed answers questions in a way in which they think the questioner wants them answered (sometimes called the **Hawthorne effect**). This sort of problem is common in evaluation surveys undertaken by researchers who are also part of the team that deliver the service being evaluated. An example of this may be the evaluation of a programme of study being carried out by the lecturers who deliver the programme!

Interviews are often felt by novice researchers to be a quick and easy way of collecting data, but in fact they are very labour intensive and require thought and preparation. Interviews also generally have to be typed up prior to analysis, adding further time to the process.

When using interviews as a data collection method, the process of knowing when enough data have been collected requires researchers to be aware of the point at which new data cease to emerge from interviews with new participants. This awareness can only come from being familiar with the content of all of the interviews as the data collection progresses. So the researcher now needs not only to conduct the interviews but also to transcribe them, or have them transcribed, and to keep their content fresh in his or her mind at all stages of the data collection process.

A further disadvantage of the interview process is that it is easy to deviate from the role of interviewer and to become the giver of information, present your own ideas and thoughts or engage in counselling activities. This is a common pitfall for many novice nurse researchers as they struggle to move from their clinical nursing role to that of a non-clinical researcher (Tod, 2006).

Powney and Watts (1987) make the ultimate observation about the disadvantages of interviews. They note that as interviews are a way of collecting talk, and because talking is a dynamic interaction, this dynamic quality is lost when attempts are made to capture the talk – as in an interview. This gets to the nub of the problem with interview data: it is very much bound up with, and to, the time in which it was recorded. There is no doubt that the same question when asked in a different way, on a different day or by a different person will elicit a different response. Talk, which is what interviews essentially are, belongs to the people involved, and it is hard to translate understanding and feeling from that moment into something that other people can fully understand.

Types of interview

We have identified some of the major features all interviews share and have looked at some of the strategies employed in interviewing. It is worth taking time now to look at some of the major groups of interview method that are used. This will help you gain insight into how they are undertaken. Although interviews are presented in the following sections as falling into one of two main types, in fact the degree of structure within the interview process is not that easily delineated. The degree of structure within any given study will lie somewhere on a continuum from completely structured to totally unstructured (Tod, 2006).

Semi-structured interviews

Semi-structured interviews are interviews in which the key questions have been decided before the interview commences. In most cases the same questions are asked, but there is freedom within the interview protocol for the researcher to explore some of the answers given. The sequence of delivery of the questions varies from interviewee to interviewee and is guided by the responses the interviewees give (Dearnley, 2005).

Semi-structured interviews are, perhaps, the mostly widely used interview method in nursing research of whatever methodology because they have the dual advantage of having some structure while allowing for more in-depth probing of the answers a respondent gives.

Semi-structured interviews can be used with any of the qualitative research methodologies that were identified in Chapter 2. Because of the degree of structure within the process of a semi-structured interview, they cannot be seen as being as exploratory as unstructured interviews, and this may limit the interpretation of the findings of research using this particular method.

Because they do not have the same degree of detailed composition as structured interviews, semi-structured interviews can present the novice researcher with quite a challenge. Interviewers conducting semi-structured interviews still need to cover the majority, if not all, of the questions in the protocol and also need to respond to some of the issues and ideas raised by the interviewee.

Unstructured interviews

Unstructured interviews are perhaps the most difficult to conduct and require some experience on the part of the researcher. They are only unstructured in so far as they do not start with lists of questions to be asked. Unstructured interviews often use what are called **topic guides**, rather than questions. Topic guides are designed to allow the interviewee to discuss their thoughts, feeling and perceptions on a topic as they see it. They are exploratory and allow the researcher to gain insight into a topic without having formed any prior conceptions about the topic associated with a more structured list of questions.

Unstructured interviews set out to gain an in-depth view of a topic from the point of view of the interviewee and therefore use probing questioning. A key technique used is to mirror back what the individual has said in order to ensure that it has been fully understood. Commonly, the interviewer will ask the interviewee questions such as 'What did you mean when you said x?' and 'How did that make you feel?' Such questions are designed to gain more in-depth responses from the interviewee without providing any clues or guidance about what, if anything, it is that the interviewer expects to hear.

Unstructured interviews are often used in studies that seek to gain an insight into a subject about which little is known. The data they produce may then be used in the design of subsequent studies or more structured interviews on the same topic area. Because of their usefulness in studying issues, ideas and experiences about which little is known, unstructured interviews are often used in more exploratory research such as phenomenology and grounded theory.

Focus groups

Focus groups are widely used to identify consensus feelings about the provision of services and the quality of products in both the public and private sector. Focus groups are a powerful and fairly rapid way of gaining insight into the collective views of a group of people. The researcher can access the views of many individuals in one setting during what is essentially a mass interview.

A well-run focus group will gain access to the views of all of the participants and will not only uncover pre-existing ideas, feelings etc., but also collect data on how the group's discussion and interaction changed the thoughts of the group about the topic under discussion. In this way they differ slightly from interviews because the process of the focus group can lead to the individuals involved changing their views because of what other people are saying. This change in views is not something usually associated with the one-to-one interview and is something the researcher needs to take into account both when designing and when interpreting a study using the focus group method.

The internet provides opportunities for researchers to undertake focus groups in the virtual environment. There are two key approaches to focus group data collection online. The first uses a simultaneous online chatroom-like format that allows people to participate in real time, while the other is more of a discussion board format where participants can log in and comment at a time and in a place convenient to them over a set period of time. There are several advantages with the accessibility of these types of internet-based studies, not least of which is that they are cheap and can recruit a lot of people with limited effort. They are, however, hard to moderate, and if the subject matter is evocative, it is hard to lend support to the participants in a meaningful way should they become upset.

Key features

In health and social care research, face-to-face focus groups usually consist of between 6 and 12 people. Six is considered to be the minimum number of participants to enable a significant discussion while 12 is close to the maximum that will allow the whole group to participate meaningfully in the discussion. The group is brought together because they all share some characteristic or experience in common that means they can usefully discuss the issue in question.

Focus group discussions are a good way of getting rich data about the views and opinions of the individuals involved. These views and opinions may evolve and change through the course of the focus group, allowing the individuals to develop a more in-depth understanding or opinion of the topic of interest. The use of the group interview allows the participants to moderate each other's opinions and ideas through discussion, and may lead some of the participants to a point where they have a better understanding and more informed opinion of a topic than they would had they been interviewed alone. In many cases the effects of the group interaction are as interesting as the results of the focus group itself.

It is usual within focus group interviews to have one moderator, or facilitator, and one co-facilitator (also called an observer). The role of the facilitator is to keep the discussion focused on the topic under discussion, ask the questions and try to engage all of the participants in the discussion. The observer is there to collect other data by observing the body language of the participants and taking notes about any patterns of behaviour exhibited during the focus group. Observers are often also responsible for the process of recording the focus group.

Advantages

Key among the advantages of the focus group is the fact that it allows people to be collectively interviewed in one place and at one time. While this usually does not remove the need for further focus groups or interviews as part of a study, it does mean that there is a rapid collection of data into which the researcher can tap. This means that focus groups have the potential to be a relatively inexpensive means of data collection.

In common with interview methods, focus groups are useful for collecting data from people who have limited literacy skills. The other interesting component of the focus group session is that the moderator can use the group to check their understanding of what the group has said while the group is still together. This means that the participants can be involved in the data analysis and establishing the credibility of the findings. This can happen at the end of the focus group when the moderator sums up the discussion, brings together the ideas and themes raised, and asks the group to confirm that the understanding of what they have said is correct. Alternatively, the moderator can collect together the themes and ask the participants to rank them in order of importance while they are still together. This means that as well as data collection, the focus group can also be used to start the analysis of the study.

Disadvantages

Peterson and Barron (2007) identify a number of potential problems with focus group interviewing, not least among which is getting everyone in the group involved with the discussion. There are always individuals within the group who are more confident and perhaps have more to say than the rest of the group, and their opinions then tend to rise to the forefront of the discussion. Peterson and Barron (2007) suggest using sticky notes to collect people's ideas, either collectively or individually before the focus group, and then using these as a stimulus to further discussion.

Acquiescence, or passive agreement, with the main group consensus can also be a problem within a focus group. There are two problems with a submissive group that tends to agree with what is being said because it is easier to do so than to challenge an opinion that appears to be popular. The first is that the consensus view may in fact not be the consensus; it may represent the views of the most vocal or powerful people in the group. The second problem is that the researcher also wants to hear and understand minority views and opinions in order to gain a more complete insight into the topic being studied.

The issues of acquiescence and non-involvement can both be designed out by carefully selecting focus groups that consist of people with similar degrees of power – within an organisation, for instance. A good example of keeping the power of the groups even would be using separate staff and patient focus groups to investigate feelings about changes to service provision within a hospital department.

There are also problems associated with the technology needed to capture all of the data produced in the focus group setting. While in an interview it is easy to place a voice recorder between the interviewer and interviewee, in the focus group setting this is not so easy. The recording of a group conversation is not only technically difficult; it can be difficult to decipher what is being said if more than one person talks at once. It may also be hard to catch the quieter members of the group.

Transcription has the potential to change the meaning of what is said in either the focus group or interview setting. Although the interviewer should be able to ascribe meaning to comments made in the one-to-one setting, this can be quite hard to do in the focus group as different words have different meanings depending on the context and intonation used at the time of speaking. Writing up the body image and capturing the gestures and eye contact within the group is an important role of the co-facilitator as this allows such notes to be transposed on to (added to) the typed transcript of the focus group.

Observation

Observation may seem to be an unusual way of collecting data for research. Observation is something we associate with our day-to-day lives and also with the surveillance of patients in the clinical setting. Observation is, however, a powerful data collection method, and the ways in which it is undertaken, the amount of time it is undertaken for, and the location in which the observation takes place have a large impact on the outputs from the research process.

The process of data collection using observation is not unique to qualitative research. Observation is used in quantitative research, but there it tends to be more structured than in the qualitative methodologies. The things to be observed and noted are decided before the observation begins. What counts as an event for the observation is predetermined, and the data collected during the observation are ready for analysis as soon as the predetermined period and number of observations are complete.

There are a number of forms that observation can take when collecting qualitative data. The most usual form is that of participant observation, which occurs in a number of guises and is discussed in more detail below.

Participant observation

Key features

Participant observation was introduced in Chapter 2 as a method associated primarily with ethnographic research. Participant observation is exactly what it says it is – the observations a researcher makes while participating in the life of a group. The first step in the participant observation process is the identification of the question or issue to be investigated, together with some thought about how the issues to be investigated might be observed. For example, if a researcher wants to understand what influences the activities of a group of nurses working in a given setting, the observer must first have some idea of what the activities they undertake are, and how often they undertake them, where and when.

> **Concept summary: participant observation**
>
> Think about what you know about being a nurse. Consider the ideas and thoughts about what it is to be a nurse that you had before you started nursing. Now compare these ideas to the reality of actually being a nurse, or student nurse. What you will notice is that your ideas of what it means to be a nurse have changed because of your experience. They will have become more concrete and your understanding of the role of the nurse much firmer. This is similar to engaging in participant observation where participating in the life of a group increases understanding of not only what the group does but also the values and norms that the group has.

The next role for the participant observer is to gain access to the area they want to observe. This is often via what are called gatekeepers – individuals who are part of the group that the observer wants to study. Gatekeepers provide a means of accessing that group. In most cases in the health and social care sense, this will mean being honest and open about what the research is about, although explaining the full extent of the purpose of the research may change behaviours within the group.

Once within the group, the observer must decide how to undertake the observations and record what they see and hear. This can include the use of tape recording, note taking or even video recording. You may think this sounds odd in relation to observation. In this context, however, observation means not only what the researcher sees, but also what they hear and what comes to them during interviews with those being observed.

Some commentators suggest strategies and rules for participant observation that include: starting off passively, learning to fit into the group without actively seeking information; not getting too involved in what goes on; being careful to remain an observer rather than a participant and avoiding being seen as an expert on any given topic.

Field notes from observations need to be written up as soon as possible after the event to ensure that the results of the observation are fresh in the mind of the observer. Chiseri-Strater and Stone Sunstein (2006) suggest that the following data are included in all field notes:

- date, time and place of observation;
- specific facts about what happens at the site of the observation;
- sensory impressions: sights, sounds, textures, smells, tastes;
- personal, about recording field notes;
- specific words, phrases, summaries of conversations and 'insider' language;
- questions about people, or behaviours, for future investigation;
- page numbers to keep the observations in order.

It is important to identify key informants, people who are willing to talk regularly and openly to the researcher about the topics under research. These key informants are useful sources of information, but they may have their own agendas and perhaps not be representative of the group as a whole.

Statements and conversations that are made in a highly informal and voluntary manner may not be truly representative of what happens in the rest of the group or, indeed, when individuals are less aware that they are being observed or interviewed.

It is important for the observer to develop relationships with all the members of the group being observed. This may mean acting in ways similar to the group and adopting the language of the group. In many ways this is best achieved when the researcher/observer is also part of the group they are researching, for example a nurse on the ward or in the clinic that is the subject of the research. Certainly, the behaviour of an individual one-to-one with the observer may vary widely from the individual's behaviour within the group. Differences in observed behaviours are worthy of note for the researcher and add to the context and interpretation of the observation. Table 3.1 sets out five dimensions of participant observation.

As with much qualitative research, the analysis of the data collected is an ongoing process. The researcher notes the behaviours that occur and the circumstances under which they occur and creates preliminary ideas about what they are seeing and why this occurs. These ideas will take into account the behaviours and activities seen and the context within which they occur. These explanations are then subject to review during subsequent observations and data collection. These later observations may serve to support or challenge the ideas, or theories, initially generated.

Table 3.1: Five dimensions of participant observation

Role of observer	Portrayal of role to others	Portrayal of study purpose to others	Duration of research	Focus of observations
Full participant	Open	Open	Single	Narrow
Partial participant	Known to some	Partially disclosed	Several	Expanded
Onlooker	Hidden	Undisclosed/ false explanation	Long term	Very broad

Source: adapted from Patton, 1986

Advantages

The main advantage of participant observation is that it accesses many forms of potential evidence. Unlike interviews and focus groups, which are restricted to what the people involved decide to tell the researcher, observations gather additional data about what researchers notice happening. Data from the observations have a richness and thickness that potentially surpass that of the interview because they have more context, making them more closely representative of what actually happens in a given situation.

Since observation, in the qualitative sense at least, is rarely a one-off event, the researcher has the opportunity not only to collect the initial data but also to verify whether these data are a true representation of what normally happens on subsequent occasions.

Participant observation, with its associated interviews and discussions, also has the capacity not only to record what people do but also to compare what they do to what they say they do. This duality of approach allows researchers to explore the interface between feelings, thought and reality in a way that may be meaningful to the study.

Disadvantages

The fact that one individual is ascribing meaning to events that they have witnessed means that the interpretation is open to subjectivity. There are masses of data – written, recorded and in other forms – to wade through. The analysis requires a large degree of selectivity on the part of the researcher, and it may not always be obvious which data to include and which not.

There are many ethical issues associated with data collection in participant observation, not least when the observations being undertaken are covert (hidden). This raises issues around consent and autonomy, especially in the clinical setting. Patients may come and go from the hospital ward, which may mean that they are not aware of, nor have consented to, being involved in data collection for a research project even if their role in the study is only passive.

Presenting and interpreting qualitative data

The reader of research cannot be present at all of the interviews, focus groups or observations, nor can they be expected to read through all of the data collected during the study. The closest they can get to understanding the meaning of the data collected is to read the data that the researcher has analysed, interpreted and presented. Not to present the data in this way would produce a massive amount of reading, which for the casual or, indeed, diligent reader will hold limited meaning anyway. This is because even reading the transcripts of an interview does not provide an insight into the context of the conversation or of the body language that was being exhibited.

Because of the infeasibility of presenting all of the data collected within a study, certain processes and procedures need to be followed for collecting together all the data in a meaningful way for presentation to readers. This process involves identifying, whittling down and putting together the main points, observations or issues raised.

The point was made earlier that this process is open to many problems, not least of which is sifting through the data collected. The large amounts of data and their subjective nature mean that a certain amount of trust has to be placed in the choices made by the researcher about which data to present and the final interpretations.

Key features

There are a number of different approaches to the analysis of qualitative data. It is beyond the scope of this text to explore these in any detail; rather, it is important that the reader gains an insight into the overall strategies used and the reasons why they may be chosen.

As discussed in Chapter 1, the aim of qualitative research is to move from specific observations towards the generation of more general hypotheses. This process of theory generation usually occurs at the same time as the data are collected. This is quite unlike the process of data analysis that occurs in the quantitative methodologies, as we shall see in Chapter 5. Coffey and Atkinson (1996) point out that analysis is a process that pervades the whole of the qualitative research process.

The key data collected during qualitative research are the interview transcripts and the field notes, such as observations, made. The emphasis that is placed on every nuance of an interview, such as the silences, sighs and intonations, will vary according to the purpose of the research. For the most part, these relatively minor details are not an important part of data analysis. Rather, the researcher will seek to engage with the meaning of the words that the interviewee says. For observations, again the exact nature of the research question will guide the data analysis process, with most qualitative researchers choosing not to narrow the focus of their research by applying a preconceived structure.

So we are left with a great deal of data in the form of words and observations that need to be narrowed down to a form that can be presented in a useful way. The key stage in this process of moving from broad observations to a general theory is to group similar data together in some meaningful way. This is more of a creative than a scientific process, and it requires a level of judgement on the part of the researcher.

There are essentially four steps required to analyse qualitative data:

1. reducing the raw data to something more manageable;
2. filtering the important ideas out from the less significant;
3. identifying important themes;
4. constructing a theory/hypothesis or narrative account of the analysis.

Reducing the raw data to something more manageable requires the reading and re-reading of the data. For interviews and focus groups this means reading the verbatim transcripts, and for observations this means reading both narrative and observation notes. During the reading, notes are made in the margins, identifying key issues. In phenomenology these key issues are usually referred to as themes; in grounded theory they are codes; and in other qualitative research methods they come under various headings. Essentially, all qualitative analysis is about reading and identifying recurring ideas and notions from the participants.

The themes and codes identified in the first phase of the data analysis are then subjected to filtering down so that the important issues are identified and the less important removed. This filtration is not merely a matter of noting which issues occur the most times within the various interviews, focus groups and observations; it is also a matter of noting those about which people feel most strongly. Other ideas may occur quite frequently but may not hold a lot of significance for the participants, which may be reflected in the emphasis the participants place upon them.

Identification of important themes is as much an art as a science, as was suggested earlier. The important themes within a qualitative inquiry will relate at least in part to the ideas contained within the initial question. There are a number of quality management strategies that can be used within qualitative research to ensure that this process is undertaken with a degree of certainty and credibility.

- Check with the focus group/interviewee that the issues they are trying to get across have been understood by reflecting them back to them at the time of the interview.
- Send the identified themes/codes to the participants during the analysis to check if the key issues as they see them have been identified.
- Use more than one person to independently analyse the data and compare notes later.
- Be **reflexive** throughout the process and be truthful about the influences and biases of the researchers and data analysts.
- Use direct quotes and/or observations to support the themes/codes identified.
- Use qualitative data analysis software to analyse the data.

Depending on the methodology, once the themes and codes have been identified and whittled down to those that are the most important, it is time for the analyst to construct their theory or narrative account of the findings of the study, which lays bare their perception of what has been discovered. It is important that the research analysis goes beyond a mere description of the data collected, and that the analysis shows some relationship between the elements of the inquiry as identified during the study. As Patton (2002) points out, however, this process is as much about the style of the analyst as it is about intellect.

Going beyond a mere description requires that the analysis and presentation of the data manage to strike a balance between deliberate exploration of the data and open-mindedness (allowing the inductive process to lead where it will). In grounded theory this will lead the researcher to construct a theory about the issue under enquiry; in phenomenology this will result in the laying out of the key elements of the topic of interest (the essence of the phenomenon); in ethnography this will lead to an explanation of the group and how it works; and in a case study or generic qualitative research this is most likely to be a general discussion of what was found.

Once the data have been analysed, they need to be presented to the readers in a manner that allows them not only to see what the analyst has seen but also to believe it. The presentation should strike a balance between being descriptive and interpretative. There should be enough detail within the presentation to provide a deep insight into the key issues identified in the analysis. However, this needs to be tempered with enough focus, and the use of verbatim quotes, to present an argument or new theory that is believable.

Trustworthiness in qualitative research

The amount of trust that can be placed in a piece of qualitative research will depend to a great extent upon the quality of the processes that go into the data collection and the analysis (such as recording interviews and taking additional notes during a focus group). To a large degree, these rely on the description of both the data collection processes and analysis provided by the researcher that may then be judged by the reader. The idea of trustworthiness in qualitative research refers to a great extent to its ability to demonstrate both rigour (in the process of data collection; see earlier) and the **relevance** of the outcomes of the study (the quality of the product).

Henwood and Pidgeon (1992) suggest seven criteria for measuring good qualitative research; these criteria are associated with means of achieving sound research and as such provide a useful insight into how we might measure qualitative research quality.

Concept summary: qualitative research quality

1. *The importance of fit* – The themes from the analysis should fit the data: demonstrated by writing explicit accounts of how themes were derived.
2. *Integration of theory* – The relationship between the themes from the analysis and how they might be integrated (e.g. combined to generate a theory).
3. *Reflexivity* – The role of the researcher in the process is accounted for in the paper.
4. *Documentation* – An audit trail exists: the paper contains a comprehensive account of what was done and why decisions were made.
5. *Theoretical sampling and negative case analysis* – The researcher should continuously modify any emerging theory to include cases who do not fit the norm.
6. *Sensitivity to negotiated realities* – The researcher shows awareness of context, power and participant reactions within the process; especially true where there is a difference in interpretation between the research and the participants.
7. *Transferability* – Realistic suggestions about how the research findings might be usefully applied to help question and inform other related contexts of human experience.

(Adapted from Henwood and Pidgeon, 1992.)

While many of these are a matter of judgement and personal interpretation, the fact that a researcher has taken the time to address elements of quality is a positive indication of intent. For the novice reader, or doer, of qualitative research the key indicators of quality might well be considered to be the clarity with which the processes are explained and the degree to which the suggested findings are seen to fit (or perhaps coherently challenge) their pre-existing view of reality.

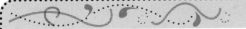

Chapter summary

This chapter has presented some of the methods used in the collection of data in qualitative research. We have seen that the collection of verbal data for qualitative research has both great advantages and disadvantages, and that whether data are collected via interview or focus group, the process needs to be carefully managed. We have also noted that observation is an important tool of data collection in qualitative research, which involves the researchers themselves being tools of data collection.

We have seen that qualitative research methods produce data that are very subjective in nature and that require the adoption of careful processes in order to add credibility and rigour to the qualitative research process. Key to the selection and execution of the data collection method within a qualitative inquiry is to understand the nature of the question that the research has set out to answer and what might be the best way of accessing that information.

We have seen that the nature of qualitative data collection is such that it is produced in large quantities that require careful collation and management. We have also seen that the process of data analysis in qualitative research involves extracting meaningful insights that contribute to the development of new understanding. This means that the qualitative researcher has to make a number of decisions about how they will analyse and present the data they have collected, and be able to justify these decisions.

Activities: Brief outline answers

Activity 3.1: Reflection (page 48)

Barriers that exist to good communication in the busy ward setting include the presence of other people and the inability of most ward areas to be able to provide privacy for such conversations to take place. Within the care setting, issues of time, the use of professional language and power relationships can also be barriers to good communication.

Activity 3.2: Research and finding out (page 50)

A great deal of human communication is non-verbal. That is, much communication is expressed in body language (for example, the way people hold their bodies, eye contact, smiling). In the case of verbally recorded interviews, it is not possible to capture this non-verbal communication unless the interviewer writes timed notes about posture and facial expressions at different points in the interview process.

Further reading

Curtis, EA and Redmond, R (2007) Focus groups in nursing research. *Nurse Researcher.* 14 (2): 25–37.

A short and useful introduction to the background and pros and cons of focus group in research, with examples.

Kvale, S and Brinkmann, S (2008) *InterViews: Learning the craft of qualitative research interviewing*, 2nd edn. London: Sage.

A comprehensive guide to interviews.

Polit, DF and Beck, CT (2008) *Nursing research: generating and assessing evidence for nursing practice* (8th edn). London: Wolters Kluwer/Lippincott Williams & Wilkins.

Part Five (Analyzing and interpreting research data) provides a quality discussion of data analysis.

Useful websites

http://onlineqda.hud.ac.uk/Intro_QDA/what_is_qda.php A short but useful introduction to qualitative data analysis.

http://onlineqda.hud.ac.uk/Intro_QDA/phpechopage_titleOnlineQDA-Examples_ QDA.php Examples of qualitative data analysis.

http://sru.soc.surrey.ac.uk/SRU19.html An overview of focus group research.

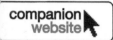

For further activities and other useful material, visit the companion website at **www.sagepub.co.uk/ellis_research2e**

Chapter 4
Overview of quantitative methodologies

NMC Standards for Pre-registration Nursing Education

This chapter will address the following competencies:

Domain 1: Professional values

9. All nurses must appreciate the value of evidence in practice, be able to understand and appraise research, apply relevant theory and research findings to their work, and identify areas for further investigation.

Domain 3: Nursing practice and decision-making

1. All nurses must use up-to-date knowledge and evidence to assess, plan, deliver and evaluate care, communicate findings, influence change and promote health and best practice. They must make person-centred, evidence-based judgments and decisions, in partnership with others involved in the care process, to ensure high quality care.
10. All nurses must evaluate their care to improve clinical decision-making, quality and outcomes, using a range of methods, amending the plan of care, where necessary, and communicating changes to others.

NMC Essential Skills Clusters

This chapter will address the following ESCs:

Organisational aspects of care

9. People can trust the newly registered graduate nurse to treat them as partners and work with them to make a holistic and systematic assessment of their needs; to develop a personalised plan that is based on mutual understanding and respect for their individual situation promoting health and well-being and minimising risk of harm and promoting their safety at all times.

For entry to the register:

14. Applies research based evidence to practice.
16. People can trust the newly registered graduate nurse to safely lead, co-ordinate and manage care.

For entry to the register:

2. Takes decisions and is able to answer for these decisions when required.
3. Bases decisions on evidence and uses experience to guide decision-making.

Introduction

Dr John Snow was credited with undertaking the first major **epidemiological** study in 1854. An outbreak of cholera (an infectious diarrhoea illness) was affecting and killing a large number of people living in the Soho area of London, England. At that time, it was widely believed that miasmas (invisible and infected vapours carried on the wind) were the cause of ill health and disease; bacteria and viruses had not yet been discovered. Snow mapped the homes of the people affected by the disease and was drawn to believe (although he had no medical reason for believing this) that a water pump on Broad Street was the source of the outbreak. Snow persuaded the city authorities to remove the handle from the pump so that no water could be drawn from it and the number of infections and deaths fell away rapidly.

Epidemiology is the study of causes and consequences of disease in populations and is widely regarded as the major scientific discipline underpinning the practice of evidence-based medicine. For the most part, epidemiological studies are quantitative and employ fairly rigid and well-defined rules to ensure the accuracy of their findings. This chapter introduces you to the major quantitative methodologies (which are often termed epidemiological methodologies) and explains the theoretical and practical differences between them. It identifies the sorts of questions that quantitative methodologies can be used to explore and the key characteristics of quantitative research. It then examines some of the main methodologies you will encounter in your nursing education and beyond. These are: quasi-experimental and experimental studies/randomised controlled trials; cohort studies; case-control studies and cross-sectional studies.

The chapter explores the strengths and weaknesses of each of these methodologies and considers which methodologies would be most suitable for different types of research question. For example, when the research is seeking to prove causality (i.e. demonstrating cause and effect as in exposure to asbestos causing mesothelioma or vaccination against the human papilloma virus reducing the risk of cervical cancer), then only methodologies accepted to prove cause and effect (i.e. experimental and cohort studies) can be used. Other methodologies (case-control and cross-sectional) can be used to explore potential associations between a cause and effect (e.g. to explore a potential, but unproven link between mobile phone use and brain tumours) but are not regarded as sufficiently scientific to prove causality. The chapter also looks at the sampling methods (i.e. the ways in which study subjects are chosen) that can be used for each of the research methodologies identified.

The knowledge you gain from this chapter will enable you to identify quantitative research when you come across it in your own reading, and to evaluate and understand the methodologies used. It will also enable you to start thinking about how you could use these research methodologies to improve your own practice especially after registration, as highlighted in the NMC Standards and Essential Skills Clusters identified at the start of the chapter.

Key characteristics of quantitative research

Quantitative research methodologies are used to answer questions that have a numerical element to them, or that set out to prove an association between two variables (cause and effect). Essentially, quantitative methodologies fall into one of two broad classifications: those that are **interventional** (or **experimental**) and those that are **observational**. Interventional studies seek to manipulate an exposure (the **independent variable**) in order to measure what effect it has on an outcome (the **dependent variable**). For example, increasing education for people with diabetes (the independent variable or **exposure**) to improve their blood glucose levels (the dependent variable or **outcome**). Observational studies, on the other hand, seek to explore the associations between a naturally occurring independent variable (exposure) and a dependent variable (outcome) (Gordis, 2008). This is because it is simply not always possible to be certain about what has caused something, often because there may be several potential causes contributing to an effect, some of which are known about and some of which are not, and it is necessary, therefore, to be more cautious about assigning a 'cause'. The terms **association** or sometimes **correlation** (although this also has a strict research meaning, as you will see in the Glossary) are used instead. For example, there is an association between being obese (the independent variable or exposure) and developing type 2 diabetes (the dependent variable or outcome), but the development of type 2 diabetes is also associated with a family history of the disease and other environmental and lifestyle factors.

Concept summary: cause and effect

A cause is simply something that has an effect. In quantitative research terminology it is common for a number of terms to be used for cause and effect, but essentially quantitative research is interested in causes (independent variables or exposures) and effects (dependent variables or outcomes). So we could describe the same event in one of three ways.

1. A nosebleed (effect) may result from a punch to the nose (cause).
2. A nosebleed (dependent variable) may result from a punch to the nose (independent variable).
3. A nosebleed (outcome) may result from a punch to the nose (exposure).

The dependent variable is best thought of as occurring only if the independent variable has occurred. In this case the nosebleed is dependent on there having been a punch to the nose – had the punch not been thrown, the nosebleed would not have happened. The independent variable is not affected by the dependent variable – quite obviously, a nosebleed will not cause a punch on the nose!

Understanding independent and dependent variables

This may all seem a bit complicated, but it is essentially just the terminology and rules that are applied to the study of cause and effect in healthcare. Understanding the nature and realities of cause and effect allows nurses and other health professionals to intervene in a meaningful way in the lives of their patients. For example, having an understanding of the fact that smoking causes coronary heart disease, lung disease and cancers is useful for nurses who are seeking to engage in meaningful health promotion. Understanding that applying compression stockings after surgery reduces the occurrence of deep vein thromboses when compared to not using them equips nurses with information for practice that is worthwhile and potentially life-saving. Such evidence-based practice reflects a number of the NMC competencies and essential skills discussed above.

The importance of quantitative research to nursing practice is clearly established, but the fact that nurses undertake little in the way of quantitative research is of some concern. Establishing the benefits, or not, of some nursing practices would serve to advance nursing knowledge and practice and, more importantly, would be of great service to our patients. For example, using a randomised prospective study, Hoe and Nambiar (1985) demonstrated that the traditional nursing practice of shaving patients prior to surgery did not in fact reduce wound infection rates. Interestingly, a literature review by Bradshaw and Price (2007) demonstrated that the common practice of inserting rectal suppositories blunt end first – believed by many nurses to be evidence based – is based only on one questionnaire-based study published in *The Lancet* in 1991 that has not been subsequently verified!

There are a number of questions that quantitative research methods can be used to answer and, like qualitative methods, there are a number of issues that the researcher has to take heed of before attempting to design a quantitative study. The key questions that the methodologies explored in this chapter can answer are outlined in Table 4.1.

What is apparent from the table is that the sorts of questions that quantitative methodologies can answer are, in fact, highly interrelated. They tend towards asking questions about causes and effects and things that can be measured in one way or another, and they all have a numerical element to them. It is important to bear in mind, however, that if practice is to be established or changed on the basis of some quantitative research, it is imperative that the correct methodology is chosen and properly applied. Table 4.1 gives an indication of the sorts of theoretical questions that can be answered using the different approaches. What follows will expand on these and give you a deeper insight into the questions and answers that the different methodologies can be used to ask and answer, as well as the key features of these methodologies.

Table 4.1: Questions that different quantitative methodologies can be used to answer

Questions	*Methodology*
If x is done, what will happen? If x is done, how often will y happen?	Experiment/quasi-experiment/ randomised controlled trial
If a person is exposed to x, will they develop outcome (disease) y? Does exposure to x cause outcome y?	Cohort studies
What exposure x might have caused this individual to have outcome y?	Case-control studies
In this group of people how many have been exposed to x or have outcome y? What is the prevalence of x or y in this group?	Cross-sectional studies
The data show that when x increases in the population so too does y – might they be associated? When exposure x increases and outcome y increases is there potential that the two are associated in some way?	Ecological studies

---

Activity 4.1   *Reflection*

Stop and think about the area that you are currently working in or your last placement. What type of questions might quantitative research be used to answer about the sort of patient problems, or the care delivery, that is undertaken there?

There are some possible answers at the end of the chapter.

Experimental and quasi-experimental research

Key features

The type of experiment described here does not relate to experiments that take place in the laboratory, but to ones that involve the researcher (or experimenter) examining the relationship between two variables – for example, does giving sucrose reduce the perception of pain in neonates? These experiments are carried out **prospectively** (that is, data are collected in real time and do not rely on memory or old notes) in an attempt to prove cause and effect. The reason that any experiment is conducted is because there is genuine uncertainty about which treatment is best for the participants. This is called the uncertainty principle (described in Chapter 1), and 'best' in this context might be taken to mean cheapest, safest, most effective or easiest to use.

Observational studies (such as case-control and cross-sectional studies, which are studies that involve no intervention on the part of the researcher and are described later in this chapter) often lead to the generation of ideas for testing using experimental study designs. Sometimes it is hard to know which of two variables in an observational study caused the other to happen (if, indeed, they are at all related). A good example of this is the debate around the use of cold remedies. If a patient takes a cold remedy and gets better within a few days, they may think that the remedy 'cured' their cold. You might then ask the question, 'If the patient took the remedy and got better, does it matter whether the remedy worked or not?' Indeed, this is a reasonable response, but what if the remedy were toxic, expensive or potentially dangerous? Many modern medicines and treatments are expensive and many have a host of side effects, and sometimes the medication or treatment has no real effect. The question therefore becomes 'Why undertake treatments or give medications that are costly and have no benefits, or that are actually worse than doing nothing at all?'

Avoiding unnecessary expense and side effects provides one reason why it is important to undertake experimental studies into the usefulness of medications and other health-related interventions. Such questions require experimental approaches to answering them and demonstrate why these approaches are favoured in modern healthcare.

Case study

As an example of a clinical observation that was proven wrong by a randomised controlled trial, the increased risk of cardiovascular events (especially stroke) in post-menopausal women taking hormone replacement therapy (HRT) was identified only during a randomised controlled trial (RCT; an important experimental method, explained below) of HRT against a placebo (Writing Group for the Women's Health Initiative Investigators, 2002). Prior to this RCT, it had been thought that HRT actually protected women against cardiovascular events.

So experiments and quasi-experiments are types of research that are done to test cause and effect. The cause (or independent variable) is manipulated, or introduced, by the researcher under carefully controlled conditions, and the effect (or dependent variable) is then measured. Experiments and quasi-experiments are widely used to test the usefulness of: educational programmes in increasing understanding; clinical interventions in improving clinical outcomes; medicines in improving the management of disease; screening to identify disease; and the changing of methods of care delivery to improve the patient experience and satisfaction.

Hypotheses

When conducting an experiment it is good practice to start with a hypothesis. A hypothesis is quite literally an idea that is less than or below (hypo) a proposition or idea (a thesis). That is, it is an idea that has yet to be tested or proven using the scientific method. The box shows the important characteristics of a hypothesis.

> **Concept summary: a hypothesis**
>
> Critical features of a hypothesis
>
> - Suggest the relationship between the variables.
> - Identify the nature of the relationship.
> - Point to the research design to be used.
> - Indicate the population to be studied.

Hypotheses are often arrived at as the result of either experience, clinical observation or other observational research. Hypotheses remain theoretical until proven otherwise and even once 'proven' they remain open to further study.

We have seen that in an experimental study the researcher manipulates one or more independent variables to see what happens to the dependent variable. In their simplest form (see Figure 4.1) this means manipulating one independent variable in one group of participants and measuring the change in a dependent variable (often called a pre-post-test or before-and-after study).

Weaknesses

There are a number of issues with this type of study, not least of which is that there is nothing to compare the intervention to and the outcome (reduced muscle pain in the example in Figure 4.1) might have occurred anyway if the person had just been left alone. Or perhaps it was the attention being paid to the individual that reduced their pain, and not the massage itself. The first issue is an example of what is called a **temporal effect**. This means it is an effect that occurs over time. The second issue is an example of the **placebo effect** – a perceived or measurable improvement in a person's condition that is not due to any active intervention but is, rather, the result of what is probably a subconscious psychological response to having an intervention (Hennekens and Buring, 1987).

There are two other issues with this type of simple experimental design: first, regression to the mean and second, testing effects. Regression to the mean occurs when individuals who have a

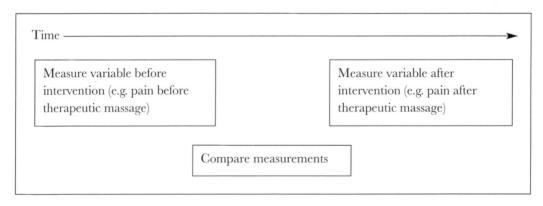

Figure 4.1: A simple experimental design

variable measured for a second time in the post-test tend towards measurements that are more average than they were on the first occasion (e.g. satisfaction scores increase in those with initially low scores and decrease a little in those with initially high scores). This may happen regardless of the effects of the intervention (Bland and Altman, 1994). The other problem that may occur in this type of experiment results from the effects of the testing itself. For example, people subjected to a test involving an educational intervention may go away from the pre-test and find out about gaps in their knowledge, so when they are retested after the educational intervention their scores will rise because of the combined effects of the education and their own research. One way to overcome this is to do the pre- and post-tests a long way apart; the other is to introduce a **control arm** to the experiment (see randomised controlled trials, pages 73–5).

Quasi-experiments

The term quasi-experiment can be applied to the observation and measurement of changes that occur naturally (sometimes called natural experiments). Raanaas et al. (2012) studied the effects of having a view of nature through a window in a residential rehabilitation programme on the physical and mental well-being of residents. They found that having an unobstructed view (independent variable) had a positive effect on self-reported physical and mental well-being. Patients in this study were randomly allocated as is usual practice in the centre. It may seem odd to think that this is an example of an experiment, because there is no manipulation of any variable by the researcher. However, when you consider that it might be impossible, or unethical, to undertake experiments on many subjects/issues (for example, denying an individual a view from their room for the purposes of the study alone), then the benefits of the natural experiment become more apparent. Figure 4.2 represents a quasi-experimental design diagrammatically.

A second form of quasi-experiment takes the methodology a little further. It examines two unrelated groups of people between which there is some difference in an independent variable. Measures are then taken of a suspected dependent variable, and the dependent variable for the two groups or fixed cohorts is compared. For example, Pesonen et al. (2007) report increased depressive symptoms in adults who had been evacuated from home during the Second World War as opposed to those who had not. The independent variable here is the evacuation (or not) and the dependent variable is depression. These are also called natural experiments comparing two fixed cohorts.

The third variation of the quasi-experiment is the pre-test post-test, such as the study by Starc and Strel (2012), which examined levels of fitness in children before and after the implementation of a new Physical Education programme delivered by specialist PE teachers. In this form of quasi-experiment the subjects effectively become their own controls (see control arm in the Glossary). This design of quasi-experiment is very useful in health policy research as it allows researchers to gauge the effectiveness of new healthcare policies on whole populations without disadvantaging any groups.

Quasi-experiments rely solely, therefore, on the measurement of unmanipulated independent and dependent variables. Because of this, and because there is no control over the environment in which the study takes place, there is a real danger that the outcomes of such experiments are affected by factors that are unknown to the researcher, and the result of such experiments therefore need to be treated with great caution. When working with such data, there is a real need to be certain that there is some plausibility to the associations being made!

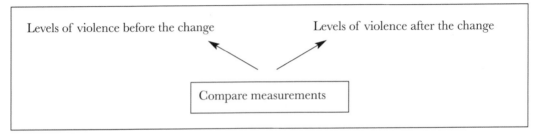

Figure 4.2: A quasi-experimental (natural experiment) design

Sampling in experimental and quasi-experimental research

The sample (that is, the individuals to be studied) chosen for an experimental study depends on the question posed in the hypothesis. Take the example of therapeutic massage and pain relief in Figure 4.1. First, it is important to define what constitutes pain and what part of the body is affected – let us say muscle pain in the thigh following sporting injury. There is a need to sample people from the population that exist with this condition, but there may well be a need to be more precise in defining the sample so that the effects of massage in a well-defined group are actually measured and described. The research sample may therefore consist of people experiencing a first soft tissue injury of the leg with no broken bones. The outcome of the study would therefore apply only to people with the identified and described injury and not to other people experiencing a similar injury in their shoulder, say, or to people experiencing a second injury to the same thigh muscles. Figure 4.3 gives a diagrammatic representation of sampling.

Once these criteria are met and a large population (that is, people with the relevant injury) is identified, individuals for the study may then be chosen from that population – this is called the study sample. When the selection process gives everyone in the larger population the same chance of being in the study (so long as they meet the other criteria), this is called **probability sampling**, and when the sample size is big enough (often calculated using statistical formulae), a sample that is **representative** of the larger population has been produced.

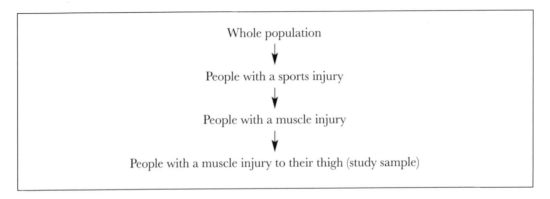

Figure 4.3: Sampling within an experimental study

Activity 4.2   *Research and finding out*

Look up and write down a definition of representativeness in research. Keep the definition to hand.

There is a specimen answer given at the end of the chapter.

In a natural experiment, the sample for the study is quite plainly the people who have experienced the phenomenon that is being researched. In the simple natural experiment they are the whole population affected by the change, while in the fixed cohorts design they are chosen because they come from one or other of the two groups under study.

Methods used in data collection

Data collection in experimental and quasi-experimental studies depends on the exact question being investigated. The data collected can include: data about the independent variable, such as demographic data (such as age, gender and ethnicity), which may be collected from pre-existing sources such as databases or from individuals themselves; data on a phenomenon (such as a sports injury or natural disaster), which may exist in patient notes, be collected from news sources or be collected especially for the study by interview or questionnaire (as with the data about evacuation during the Second World War by Pesonen et al. (2007), discussed above). Outcome (dependent variable) data may also be collected from existing records or may be specially collected for the study using data collection methods such as interviews, questionnaires, physical examination or biological samples. For example, Pesonen et al. (2007) used an established questionnaire (the Beck Depression Inventory) to measure the presence of depression in their study.

Randomised controlled trials

Key features

Randomised controlled trials (RCTs) are widely considered to be the 'gold standard of proof' for a clinical intervention or the effectiveness of a medication. RCTs are conducted in a specific manner so that they are capable of answering a very specific question, or set of interrelated questions, for example: to determine the effectiveness of acupuncture, versus sham acupuncture; to reduce the anxiety some women experience when undergoing in vitro fertilisation (IVF) treatment (Isoyama et al., 2012); to compare the differences in plasma sodium levels following major surgery in children prescribed either Hartmann's solution and 5% dextrose or 0.45% saline and 5% dextrose (Coulthard et al., 2012); and to determine which is the better treatment regimen for people with newly diagnosed dementia – GP care or dementia clinic care (Meeuwsen et al., 2012). You may want to look up some of these in the library or online and explore how they have been undertaken.

RCTs are a very specific application of the experimental method identified above as they use techniques to explore the relationships between two variables while maintaining direct control over other factors that may affect the **validity** and **reliability** of the findings.

> **Concept summary: validity and reliability**
>
> Validity refers to the ability of a methodology (or data collection technique) to measure what it is supposed to be measuring. For example, we know that a thermometer (if placed correctly for long enough) will measure temperature, but it is not easy to be certain that a questionnaire designed to measure quality of life actually does so, because it is not always easy to define what quality of life actually is.
>
> Reliability refers to whether a method of data collection, or a measurement, will repeatedly give the same results if used by the same person more than once or by two or more people when measuring the same phenomenon.

Because RCTs control many of the variables that a simple experiment does not, they have found favour as a source of evidence in medicine and, as the examples given above show, also in nursing circles. To understand why RCTs are so highly regarded it is worth paying attention to the key features of their design. The following discussion relates to the best possible design for an RCT. However, it should be remembered that RCTs are very often conducted in humans, so there are good practical and ethical reasons why not all RCTs contain all of the features discussed below. An example of this is the emergence over the last decade or so of more **equivalence studies**, where the current treatment for a condition is used instead of a placebo or **sham treatment** for comparison (see later) because it would be unethical not to treat people in the control arm. A control arm for a study provides the researchers with a group of individuals whose outcomes can be compared to the outcomes for the individuals in the study arm. People in the control arm of a study are treated in an identical manner to people in the study arm of the study minus the intervention or drug being tested. By doing this, the researcher can be sure that it is the intervention or the drug being researched that has caused the outcome of interest and not merely the fact that the individual has been involved in a research study.

RCTs are always conducted in a prospective manner, which, as was discussed earlier in this chapter, means that data are collected in real time and do not rely on participant recall or old notes or data. The study question is sometimes posed as a hypothesis, and sometimes as a **null hypothesis** (or the opposite of the outcome that the researchers expect to see and what the study sets out to disprove). The reasons for this relate to the statistics that the study team will use and are not of great significance here. RCTs use one group on which a new intervention is tried and at least one other group on which the new intervention is not tried and with which the first group are compared. Both groups are treated in the same way, other than the intervention (the independent variable), so that the people conducting the RCT can demonstrate that the intervention, and nothing else, has caused the differences in outcomes (the dependent variable) between the groups. This is why they are an improvement on the simple experimental methodology described earlier. Figure 4.4 gives a diagrammatic representation of a simple RCT design.

Case (gets the intervention being investigated)

Time ———————————————————→ Outcome(s) of interest measured

Direction of enquiry —————————————→

Control (does not get the intervention being investigated)

Figure 4.4: A simple RCT design with one control group

Activity 4.3   *Research and finding out*

You may like to find out if any RCTs are, or have been, undertaken where you are currently on placement. Find out if there is a research nurse attached to the department you are working in and see whether they would be happy to discuss any current projects with you. If there are no examples for you to draw upon, reflect on your activities during the course of the day and try to identify an area in which you think there might be a good argument for undertaking an RCT. What do you think might be the problems with trying to undertake an RCT in a clinical setting?

There are some possible answers at the end of the chapter.

Sampling in RCTs

The first problem with the above method, if we take it at face value, is whether the two groups (cases and controls) are actually alike at the start of the study. The simple solution to this question might seem to be matching the two groups up for all the things that we can measure to make sure that they are alike. So, for example, if we wanted to test the usefulness of a new drug for lowering high blood cholesterol levels, we could get together a group of people who had high cholesterol and then split it into two groups. We could make sure that the two groups were evenly matched for ages, gender, ethnicity, body mass index, whether they had high blood pressure or diabetes, etc., and claim that the two groups starting the study were identical. Indeed, if we accept that the issues identified are important in determining how people might respond to the drug this might seem reasonable. Some studies do closely match cases and controls for known variables, usually because there are few participants available for the research and sample sizes are small.

Matching cases and controls for all known variables is not always a good idea, since what this approach does not necessarily do is split the variables that we cannot see or measure – for instance, participant attitude and likely adherence to the trial regime, genetic make-up, social criteria, diet – evenly between the two groups. It is quite conceivable that these criteria are unevenly distributed among the participants and are affected by criteria we do not yet know about and lack the ability to measure. So the more usual way of dealing with the creation of the two groups is to allow them to be generated randomly, often by a computer or randomisation table.

The study starts with participants that all meet the inclusion criteria and are therefore similar in a number of ways. They are then randomly split into two groups so that variables that can be seen and measured and variables that cannot be seen and measured are likely to be split evenly between the two groups (assuming that the number of participants included in the trial is large enough).

There is another reason that study staff do not split the participants into the two groups themselves, and this is called **selection bias**. Selection bias occurs when a researcher places a person in one arm of the study because they believe, perhaps subconsciously, that the person will benefit the most from the new intervention and/or that they are likely to show the new intervention in its best light.

Activity 4.4   *Critical thinking*

Imagine that you are involved in an RCT and are responsible for recruiting participants to the study and allocating them to be either cases or controls. Obviously you want the study to be a resounding success. What factors might affect the way in which you allocate people, assuming you have the choice about which arm of the study to put them into?

There are some possible answers at the end of the chapter.

The study is now at the point where the two groups have been determined and the new intervention is being applied in the case group and not in the control group. This gives rise to two new questions: 'Does it matter if the participant can tell which group they are in?' and 'Does it matter if the researcher can tell which group each participant is in?'

Blinding in RCTs

The simple answer to these questions is that it is preferable that neither the participant nor the researcher can tell which group any individual participant is in. There are some good reasons for this. Participants are known to react differently if they know they are getting a new intervention. Returning to the cholesterol-lowering drug example, if the participants know they are on the cholesterol-lowering drug, they may choose to be less careful about their diet because, after all, they are getting the real thing; conversely, they may choose to increase their exercise and improve their diet because they want the study to work. Such **behavioural biases** (called the Hawthorne effect) will affect the confidence that can be placed in the study findings.

Activity 4.5   *Communication*

Next time you are on placement try this simple exercise: greet half of your patients and colleagues by saying 'Alright!' and the other half by saying 'How are you?' Note the types of responses that you get. Why do you think the responses differ?

There is an explanation of this activity at the end of the chapter.

If the researcher knows what arm of a study a participant is in, this too may change their behaviour, either consciously or subconsciously, again because they want to be part of something that succeeds. This may mean that in a trial of a new wound dressing they report improved wound healing for a new dressing; or in the cholesterol lowering example, they may give the intervention group more education about diet, exercise and smoking cessation than they give to the control group.

To avoid behavioural biases, the best RCTs blind both the participants and the researcher to which arm of the study each participant is on. This **blinding** (now sometimes called **masking**) is usually achieved by the use of a placebo in a drug trial or a sham intervention in a trial of a treatment. A placebo is a drug that looks exactly like the drug being trialled, but that does not contain the active drug. Sham interventions are harder to provide; for instance, it is hard to pretend to give therapeutic massage or to hide which wound dressing is being used. One way round this is for the person delivering the intervention and the person recording the effectiveness of the intervention to be different so that prior knowledge of what treatment a patient is receiving does not **bias** the measurements being taken.

Methods used for data collection

RCTs use a number of methods for collecting the study data. These methods include clinical and non-clinical measurements (e.g. blood cholesterol levels, wound healing rates, participant satisfaction and quality of life data). The methods used for data collection are determined by the outcomes that the study is measuring. All methods of data collection need to measure the variables concerned both accurately and clearly (Macnee and McCabe, 2008). This means that when designing research it is important to define what is being measured as well as how it is being measured, by whom and when, and to ensure that all researchers involved in the study (which may be taking place across many different sites, for example) follow precisely the same protocol.

Many RCTs collect data on more than one outcome, so they may use clinical measures and questionnaires simultaneously to obtain data to answer the research question. In order to maintain blinding, the results of clinical tests such as cholesterol levels are not known to either the researcher or the participant but are surveyed by a monitoring team who also have responsibility for making sure that the participants in a study are kept safe and that a study is stopped if there are any unforeseen adverse consequences.

Many of the questionnaires used in RCTs and other forms of quantitative research have been previously validated, that is, they have been tested on many occasions in several groups of individuals to make sure that the questions they contain give a true picture of what people actually think or feel about an issue. A common example of such a questionnaire is the Short Form 36 (SF36), which is used to measure an individual's health and well-being, as they see it (www.sf-36.org).

Cohort studies

Key features

Cohort studies are usually prospective and follow a predetermined group of individuals through time and measure the **incidence** of predetermined outcomes. For example, cohort studies might be used to follow a group of workers in the asbestos industry for a period of years to determine the incidence of mesothelioma (a type of lung cancer associated with exposure to asbestos) in that group (Nicholson et al., 1982). The purpose of cohort studies is to link an exposure (independent variable or cause – in this case, asbestos) with an outcome (dependent variable or effect – in this case, mesothelioma). Cohort studies are said to be able to determine the causality of disease, that is, they are able to link exposure to a certain independent variable with a disease being researched.

Concept summary: cohorts

To understand the concept of cohorts, think about the people that you trained or are training with. They are your training cohort. Because you are training in a caring profession, you will share some characteristics: you are all likely to like people, be caring and hold similar political and social views. Because you are training or have trained together, you share similar skills because you have been exposed to similar classroom and clinical situations. As you are a cohort, it is likely therefore that you will have some shared outcomes that result from your shared exposures.

Unlike the experimental study designs discussed earlier, cohort studies do not involve an intervention on the part of the researcher – they are purely observational. It is the fact that these studies are undertaken prospectively and that they explain the biological reasons for the disease outcome that makes them able to determine the causality of disease. Figure 4.5 gives a diagrammatic representation of a simple cohort study.

What you will notice from Figure 4.5 is that some people get the disease even though they were not thought to be exposed to a cause of the disease. There are two main reasons for this. First, disease may have more than one cause and so the cohort study provides insight into how much is actually caused by the exposure under investigation rather than other environmental or lifestyle exposures. Second, people are often exposed to things they do not know about, for example, they

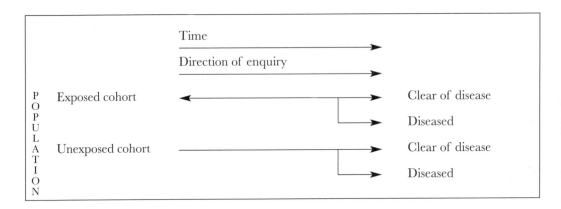

Figure 4.5: A simple cohort study design with one control group

may be exposed to asbestos in an old house or place of work.

Some cohort studies are **retrospective** in nature (that is, they look back in time) and try to collect data about an exposure (a potential cause of disease) and relate it to an outcome (often a disease). However, less faith is placed in the outcomes of these types of studies because they are not prospective and so rely on the recall of participants for things such as dietary or smoking history. This may cause **recall bias**, which leads to questions about whether the study does indeed demonstrate what it claims to demonstrate. Last (1995) gives the example of mothers of children with leukaemia being better at recalling having had X-rays while pregnant than mothers of children who do not have leukaemia when the likelihood is they have had similar numbers of X-rays.

Activity 4.6   *Reflection*

Think about one of your weaknesses – it might be chocolate, tea, alcohol or even cigarettes. Now try to remember how many/much of this weakness you had yesterday, last week, last month. When did you start? Do you always have the same quantity in a day? Are there exceptions? What are these exceptions? Have you changed brands or strengths? When? By how much?

You will see that by using just your power of recall you have to start guessing about some answers. This would lead to problems if you were trying to collect accurate data for a study!

As the answer is based on your own reflection, there is no outline answer at the end of the chapter.

As well as cohort studies that follow well-defined groups of people over a period of time to collect data on the incidence of a particular disease (as in the asbestos and mesothelioma example), there is another form of prospective cohort study design that follows people over a period of time and collects data about their lifestyle, blood pressure, diet, working lives, etc., (exposures or independent variables) as well as collecting data about the development of disease and ill health (outcomes or dependent variables) in the cohort. The data collected on exposure, and indeed non-exposure, are then compared to data on outcomes, or not, in the cohort. Inferences are then made about the causes of disease and ill health. The benefit of this form of cohort study is that it does not have to start with any preconceptions and is therefore useful in identifying causes of disease that had not previously been thought of.

There are a number of famous cohort studies that have given useful insights into what lifestyle choices, jobs, medication regimes, etc. give rise to increased likelihood of disease. Perhaps the most interesting studies for nurses are the massive and very productive Nurses' Health Studies (NHS) that are taking place in the United States (see case study box).

Case study

The Nurses' Health Study cohort research project (NHS I) was started in 1976 and its scope and cohort size were further expanded in 1989. In 1976 the study enrolled married registered nurses aged 30 to 55 who lived in the 11 US states where the state nursing boards had agreed to supply the nurses' names and addresses. Of the 170,000 nurses initially approached, approximately 122,000 nurses responded. Every two years since then, all members of the cohort have received a follow-up questionnaire regarding diseases and health-related topics, including smoking, hormone use and menopausal status. Every four years since 1980, the cohort have also received questions relating to their dietary habits, and since 1990 questions about quality of life have been added. Response rates to the questionnaires have been high, at about 90 per cent, throughout its life (www.channing.harvard.edu/nhs).

A second study (NHS II) was started in 1989 with younger participants – aged 25–42 – to study emerging areas of interest such as contraception use, diet and more lifestyle data. The cohort for this study is somewhat smaller at around 117,000 participants. NHS III is the newest study; it is web based and started to roll out in 2008, again to a younger generation of nurses.

What is interesting about these studies is that they have taken an informed set of professionals and collected data in real time over many years. If an individual nurse enrolled in 1976 and is still participating in the study – as many are – then, to date, there are approaching 40 years of data relating to the one individual. Given the size of the initial cohort, this means that the NHS I has data relating to around 4.5 million years of nurses' lives, the things they are exposed to and the outcomes and diseases these might cause. To date these studies have produced, and are still producing, approaching 300 papers relating to disease risk factors for women. Some of the key findings from the NHS I and NHS II are shown in Table 4.2. You may find that exploring the website for this study gives you some understanding of the nature of these types of study.

Table 4.2: Some of the major findings of the Nurses' Health Studies

- Birth control pills do not increase non-smoking women's risk of heart disease.
- Women who take oral contraceptives for more than five years have less than half the risk of ovarian cancer than women who have never used birth control pills.
- Women who take oestrogen after menopause decrease their risk of heart disease, but raise their risk of developing breast cancer.
- Increased dietary calcium intake among post-menopausal women is not protective against fractures of the hip and wrist, although a positive relationship has been observed between protein intake and risk of fractures.
- A diet rich in red meat raises the risk of colon cancer.
- Women who drink moderate amounts of alcohol (one to three drinks per week) cut their risk of heart attack in half, but increase their risk of breast cancer by one-third.
- Limiting fat intake and eating more high fibre foods does not reduce a woman's risk of breast cancer.
- Women who have taken multi-vitamin supplements that contain folic acid have a 75 per cent reduced risk of colon cancer.

Source: www.brighamandwomens.org/publicaffairs/NursesHealthStudy.aspx

Sampling in cohort studies

The sample selected for a cohort study is determined by the questions that the study sets out to answer. So if the study is interested in specific outcomes for a specific group (such as individuals who work with asbestos), then people who meet the criteria of interest constitute the study group or sample. If, however, the study is interested in determining several outcomes, especially where there is no suspicion of a particular disease in a group, then a more general group is chosen and followed up for a period of time, measuring a range of exposures and outcomes to see what arises (the NHS studies would fall into this category).

As with RCTs, there remains the need for a comparison group so that it is possible to compare exposure in one group to non-exposure in the other and thus determine the extent to which the outcome of interest is caused by the exposure (demonstrating causality).

There are many issues relating to how and who is selected to be in the comparison group, as there is a need to keep the two groups as alike as possible in order that the one thing that is different between the groups can be said to be the exposure that has caused the outcome. In studies such as the NHS, this is achieved by studying a large homogeneous (largely similar) group of nurses of similar ages and, when an outcome of interest arises, comparing the data on exposures between those who have the outcome (or disease) of interest and those who do not.

In more specific cohort studies, such as the asbestos workers example, the comparison group would be drawn from people who are largely similar to the group being investigated except that they are not exposed to the potential cause being investigated. So a comparison group for people who work with asbestos might include other workers in the same factory, or workers in similar jobs who live in the same communities and have broadly similar lifestyles to the group under study.

Methods used for data collection

The most frequently used data collection method in cohort studies is self-completion question-naires. The use of self-completion questionnaires is driven by the fact that these studies are so large and take place over such a long period of time that individual visits, or data collection by study staff, would be very expensive and time consuming. Some studies collect additional data from some participants for analysis of subgroups or because there is a suspicion that the extra data will yield some useful result. For example, for various purposes the NHS I has collected toenail clippings (to examine mineral content) as well as blood samples (usually more than one sample, and some years apart) from many thousands of the participants.

As with the RCT, some of the questionnaires used are previously validated while other questions and questionnaires are designed specifically for the study.

Case-control studies

Key features

Case-control studies are quite cheap and easy to do when compared with other quantitative research methods. Case-control studies are backward looking (retrospective). They study people with an outcome (or disease – the dependent variable) of interest and try to determine past exposures (the independent variable) to things that might have caused the disease (Gordis, 2008), or might predict the occurrence of an outcome. For example, Churpek et al. (2012) studied patients who had experienced a cardiac arrest in hospital and compared them to patients who had not – the predictor of interest was the Modified Early Warning Score on admission and during the 48 hours prior to the arrest; Al-Farsi et al. (2012) studied individuals with autistic spectrum disorders and matched healthy controls comparing the breastfeeding practices they had been exposed to as babies; and Martinez-Ramirez et al. (2012) compared the protein intake of elderly patients who had experienced an osteoporotic fracture and those who had not.

Case-control studies cannot be used to prove causality because they do not collect data in a prospective manner and so there are many issues relating to **confounding** and bias that may affect the quality of the data they produce. People with the disease in question may recall exposure to the causal agent better than people without the disease because they have thought about it. As explained earlier, this is called recall bias. A case-control study must have a hypothesis, or hypotheses, as this makes the design of the study easier and more understandable to people who might read it. Figure 4.6 gives a diagrammatic representation of a case-control study.

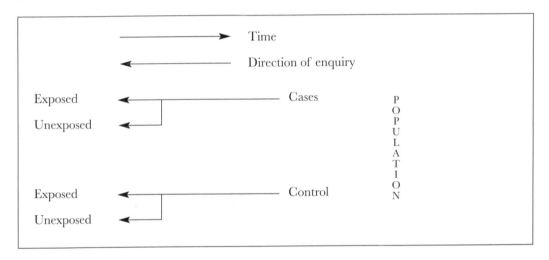

Figure 4.6: A case-control study

Concept summary: confounding

Confounding occurs when alternative explanations for an outcome in a study are not accounted for. Confounding variables are always independently associated with both the exposure and the outcome being measured. For example, an increased risk of cancer of the pancreas is associated both with smoking (the independent variable being studied) and with coffee drinking (an independent variable not being studied), and smokers tend to drink more coffee than non-smokers.

In the mesothelioma cohort study, if the control group used was very different from the study group (for example, if it was composed of office workers who as such are less likely to smoke than manual workers who work with asbestos), then smoking might be responsible for making the manual workers more susceptible to mesothelioma. So the risk of getting mesothelioma from exposure to asbestos might be overestimated if the levels of smoking in the two groups were not accounted for.

Sampling in case-control studies

The sample for a case-control study is taken by selecting people who have an outcome of interest – say, lung cancer – and matching them with appropriately matched individuals who do not have the outcome of interest. Cases need to be well defined. It is not enough, for instance, to define your sample as 'people with hypertension' (high blood pressure); it is better to state what is meant by high blood pressure (e.g. 'greater than 150/85 mmHg on three consecutive occasions'). It is also important to define where the cases are from (their source), because this provides information about how representative they are of all people with the outcome of interest. At its simplest, all cases of liver cancer in one hospital in the UK may not be representative of all cases of liver cancer, especially if the hospital is in an area of high unemployment or social deprivation, for example. When subjects are drawn from **prevalent** cases (rather than incident ones) they may be different from the whole population of people with the disease. This may be because prevalence of the disease relies on people surviving with it, whereas using incident cases does not.

Concept summary: prevalent cases

Prevalent cases are people with a disease (or other outcome of interest) at a given point in time. Incident cases are new cases of a disease (or other outcome of interest) occurring during the course of the research study. So prevalent cases are existing cases and incident cases are new cases. The important issue is survival; if a study uses prevalent cases, but the disease has a high early **mortality rate**, then prevalent cases may not represent the majority of people who get the disease because many of them will have died.

Disease duration also affects the choice of prevalent or incident cases. If one is studying an outbreak of food poisoning, then one would study incident cases as the illness is short lived. But when researching chronic diseases (such as diabetes or chronic kidney disease), the choice of prevalent or incident cases is influenced more by the research question than the disease duration.

Choosing controls for case-control studies is as much a matter of judgement as it is of science. Controls need to be chosen with care. If the aim of the study is to compare like with like, then the controls need to be very similar – in all respects other than not having the disease – to the case population.

A good example that demonstrates the need for good judgement is the study of a disease that is related to alcohol. If the cases are all people who have been admitted to hospital with the alcohol-related liver disease, it may seem sensible to compare them to other people in the hospital at the same time who are of the same gender and age. There is a problem with this, however, since people who have alcohol-related accidents or alcohol-related diseases are admitted to hospital more often than people in the population as a whole with the same gender and age. So a control group chosen like this would be less like the general population from which the cases are drawn than if it was drawn from the general population.

When next in practice, you may want to take note of the number of patients you see who smoke or have a history of excessive alcohol use.

Methods used for data collection

Data collection for case-control studies is usually undertaken by studying medical, nursing and other documentary records, by interviewing (the cases and controls or their relatives) and by taking, or using existing, biological samples. One of the major problems with case-control studies – and a good reason why they are generally used to generate hypotheses that are later tested in prospective studies – is that they often rely on participant recall.

Cross-sectional studies

Key features

Cross-sectional studies are used to find out the prevalence of an outcome or exposure in a given group of individuals. They are very common in healthcare research and are quick, cheap and easy to conduct. Cross-sectional studies allow researchers to generate hypotheses that can be tested using other quantitative methods such as RCTs and cohort studies.

Surveys are a form of cross-sectional study and may be used to find out any number of things, including demographic data, the presence or absence of disease, people's opinions and the way in which people plan to vote. It is usual practice for universities to collect data on students' opinions of the modules they are studying; this is a simple cross-sectional study usually undertaken for quality monitoring (audit) purposes.

Since data on exposures and outcomes are collected simultaneously, cross-sectional studies are not good at showing the sequence of events. For example, a cross-sectional study of mental illness and unemployment would be hard to interpret since it is likely that mental illness is both a cause and effect of being unemployed. Because of this they are the weakest of the epidemiological study designs discussed in this chapter.

> **Concept summary: prevalence and incidence rate**
>
> Prevalence is the amount of a disease in a defined population at a given point in time. So if a disease lasts for life, its prevalence will continue to rise, even if the incidence rate is low, whereas for short-lived illnesses such as colds or measles the incidence rate and prevalence will be broadly similar. Often people use the two terms interchangeably, but they are not the same thing.

Cross-sectional studies usually measure one of two types of prevalence: point prevalence ('Do you have a headache at the moment?') and period prevalence ('Have you had a headache in the last week?'). For chronic diseases (diseases that last a long time – such as asthma or diabetes) there is little difference between the two measures of prevalence, while for short-lived diseases (such as a cold or a headache) the two may be vastly different.

A cross-sectional study is essentially a snapshot of a phenomenon at a point in time and cannot, therefore, be used to demonstrate the incidence of an exposure or an outcome, unlike the prospective methods discussed earlier. Unless they are focused on high-risk groups, cross-sectional studies are not very useful for studying rare diseases. Cross-sectional studies are useful for planning the delivery of a service and for estimating future need.

Some cross-sectional studies collect data on two phenomena of interest and examine whether there is an association (or correlation) between the two, although, because cross-sectional studies are not longitudinal, they are not able to demonstrate true cause and effect. One such study by Kreinin et al. (2012) sought to examine the relationship between smoking and bipolar affective disorder.

Sampling in cross-sectional studies

The sample for a cross-sectional study is usually drawn from a population in which the exposures or outcomes of interest are known to be fairly prevalent. For example, Ellis and Cairns (2001) studied the prevalence of renal disease among older people with hypertension and/or diabetes in two GP practices. The purpose of this study was to ascertain the prevalence of early renal disease in order to inform the debate about whether screening for renal disease among this population was a worthwhile exercise.

Methods used for data collection

Data for cross-sectional studies are often drawn from pre-existing data, such as blood test results, data held on hospital or GP databases, or data held by local authorities. Such data may be supplemented during the course of a study by taking biological samples, by using questionnaires or by conducting structured interviews.

Chapter summary

This chapter has described the main quantitative methodologies used in healthcare research. It has identified that the choice of study design is influenced by a number of issues that include the nature of the question being asked, whether the study is attempting to show cause and effect (experimental designs and cohort studies) or whether it is merely interested in looking for potential associations (case-control) or merely measuring the prevalence of a phenomenon (cross-sectional studies).

We have seen that the samples used in various studies have to be carefully chosen and described in order to maintain the validity of the study and that various data collection methods are used in order to generate the findings for a given research methodology.

The following chapter describes and explores in more detail the data collection methods used in quantitative research and when they might be used, as well as their strengths and weaknesses. It shows some of the methods used for describing the data found during a quantitative study and some of the statistical tests used to generate findings.

Activities: Brief outline answers

Activity 4.1: Reflection (page 68)

Here are some types of questions that quantitative research might be used to answer.

- Does keyhole surgery involve a shorter hospital stay than conventional surgery, and if so how many days are involved?
- If we give antibiotics before inserting a chest drain, are patients less likely to get an infection?
- Is patient mortality linked to the nurse–patient ratio on the ward?
- What are the social characteristics of people who develop schizophrenia?
- Does home birth result in less complication for the mother than hospital birth?

Activity 4.2: Research and finding out (page 73)

Representativeness is the extent to which the study sample is similar to the general population from which it is drawn for important variables (e.g. gender, age, ethnicity etc.). The more representative a study sample is the more likely that the findings of the study hold true in the general population (generalisability).

Activity 4.3: Research and finding out (page 75)

Randomised controlled trials are used to determine cause and effect and may be used to demonstrate the effectiveness of a drug or a therapeutic intervention. They are also used to compare new to old drugs or usual interventions. Example investigations might include the following.

- Does patient-controlled analgesia improve patient satisfaction with knee replacement surgery when compared to four-hourly injections?
- Do children admitted to the emergency department with an exacerbation of asthma respond as well to a reservoir spacing device as they do to a nebuliser?
- Do patients with arthritis report better mobility with the new drug x than they did with the old drug y?

Problems with undertaking RCTs in the practice setting include time, making sure everyone follows the trial protocol and procedures properly, and keeping accurate records of interventions.

Activity 4.4: Critical thinking (page 76)

Any researcher might be tempted to put the sickest participants into the cases arm (group) as they might show the best response. It is also possible, depending on the study, that putting the least sick participants into the cases arm might achieve the best result. There might also be the temptation to put into the cases group the most articulate participants or those considered most likely to comply or try hardest to achieve the goals of the study. Such choices may be conscious decisions or made purely subconsciously. Either way, they mean that the study would not be comparing like with like.

Activity 4.5: Communication (page 76)

Most people like to be liked; one way that people ensure that they are liked is to behave in a way that they think you want them to behave. When you say 'Alright!', what they are hearing is 'I want you to say that you are alright', but when you say 'How are you?', they hear an open question that has no suggested response so they feel more able to respond by saying how they actually feel. This is similar to the Hawthorne effect in that people are responding to what they think you want to hear, rather than saying what they actually want to say.

Further reading

Gerish, K and Lacey, A (eds) (2006) *The research process in nursing* (5th edn). Oxford: Blackwell.

See Chapter 16 on experimental research, Chapter 17 on survey methods and Chapter 24 on questionnaire design and use.

Gomm, R and Davies, C (eds) (2000) *Using evidence in health and social care.* London: Sage.

See Chapter 2 on survey designs and Chapter 3 on experimental research.

Gordis, L (2008) *Epidemiology.* (4th edn). Philadelphia PA: Saunders.

A very accessible guide to all epidemiology, especially the research designs.

Macnee, C and McCabe, S (2008) *Understanding nursing research: reading and using research in evidence-based practice.* (2nd edn). London: Wolters Kluwer/Lippincott Williams & Wilkins.

See the section in Chapter 9 on quantitative research designs.

Parahoo, K (2006) *Nursing research: principles, process and issues.* (2nd edn). London: Palgrave Macmillan.

See Chapter 3 on quantitative designs, Chapter 11 on experimental design and Chapter 13 on questionnaires.

Useful websites

www.intute.ac.uk/socialsciences Intute is a free online service providing you with a database of hand selected web resources for education and research. This URL provides links to many websites about quantitative study designs if you type 'quantitative research health' into the search box.

www.medicine.ox.ac.uk/bandolier This is an online evidence-based medicine journal. The glossary, extended essays and the new learning zone are of great use to students of research.

www.socialresearchmethods.net/kb The Research Methods Knowledge Base is a comprehensive web-based textbook that addresses all of the topics in a typical introductory undergraduate or graduate course in social research methods. The section on experimental and quasi-experimental design is quite useful.

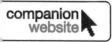

For further activities and other useful material, visit the companion website at **www.sagepub.co.uk/ellis_research2e**

Chapter 5
Data collection methods and analysis in quantitative research

> **Chapter aims**
>
> After reading this chapter, you will be able to:
>
> - identify the major data collection methods employed in quantitative research in nursing;
> - describe the advantages and disadvantages of the data collection methods used in quantitative research;
> - describe the key elements of data analysis in quantitative research;
> - demonstrate awareness of the quality issues related to data management in quantitative research.

Introduction

In the previous chapter, quantitative research methodologies were identified as a means of answering questions about cause and effect as well as correlations and associations between variables. This chapter identifies the main data collection methods used within quantitative research in nursing and explains how they meet the aims of the chosen methodology. It explores how data are collected and the pros and cons of the approaches, and it examines the use of surveys and questionnaires as data collection methods.

This chapter also looks at data presentation and data analysis in quantitative research and what they serve to demonstrate. It uses examples from the literature and some activities to demonstrate the approach to the reader in a meaningful way. It also illuminates some of the ways in which the process of data presentation and analysis in the quantitative methodologies can be demonstrated to be valid and reliable.

The aim of this chapter is not to provide an exhaustive account of the data collection methods used in quantitative research but rather to present a summary of the main methods used and the reasoning behind the processes and procedures adopted.

Key features

It is clear that the quantitative methodologies are concerned with numbers, with understanding associations between variables and with demonstrating cause and effect. Gathering such data requires researchers to engage in much thought not only about what they want to collect but also about how they might collect it and how they might ensure the quality of the process.

The key feature of all quantitative study methods is the consistency and accuracy of the data collection process. The consistency (reliability) and accuracy (validity) of the data collection ensure that the data collected are suitable to be used to generate findings that can be generalised. Unlike qualitative research, which moves from the specific observation towards the generation of more general hypotheses, the purpose of quantitative research is to move from general observations to the generation of more specific outcomes. The specific and well-defined nature of the outcome measures (the research findings) means that the results of quantitative research are often capable of being generalised (that is, applied with a fair degree of certainty outside of the research setting).

Concept summary: generalisability

Generalisability is an important feature of quantitative research because it allows the researcher to have a fair degree of certainty that the findings of the research apply to people that have the same, or broadly similar, characteristics as the people involved in the study.

Think of it this way: as nurses working in the clinical setting it is important that we feel the care we deliver to a patient will work. For example, it is important for us to know that the dressing that we apply to a particular wound or the ways in which we prevent the formation of pressure sores are going to be effective. This knowledge is generated by research that has been carried out to demonstrate this. That research has involved people who are broadly similar to the patients we care for, so we have some certainty that the information we apply from the research will be relevant to our patients.

Research into the treatment of postnatal depression applies to people with postnatal depression. The same research will not apply to the treatment of people with depression of a different aetiology (cause) or different type. The research may have taken place in only 100 people with postnatal depression, but it applies to all patients with postnatal depression who are broadly similar to the people who took part in the research. The research is generalisable to people with postnatal depression and only those people.

Nurses are familiar with undertaking treatments and care regimes that are broadly similar and that work when we apply them time and again to different patients. Such regimens are often the product of quantitative research that informs the provision of care, the outcomes of which are broadly speaking predictable. This is the first and most important premise of quantitative study design: it informs future practice. As such, it is easy to see how quantitative research might reflect the aspirations of the Nursing and Midwifery Council's (NMC) competencies and ESCs (NMC, 2010). These include using research to underpin nursing practice, as well as using research to evaluate the quality of the care that is currently provided.

When discussing the qualitative methodologies, we saw that the researcher is seen as a tool of data collection and that this provides a depth and richness to the process. This personal engagement with the collection of data was identified as necessary to the need to understand the human interactions that form the basis of qualitative research. We also identified that, because of the interactive nature of the data collecting methods in qualitative research, it is hard to eradicate bias in qualitative research.

The collection of data within the quantitative methodologies requires researchers to be one step removed from the process, so they remain objective and their approach to the process is consistent. This detachment ensures that the quality of the data collected is high and there is less room for bias (the introduction of systematic errors) to creep into the data collection process.

The rest of the chapter explores the use of the quantitative data collection methods that are most commonly used in nursing research: questionnaires, surveys, structured interviews and the collection of clinical (physiological) data. In order to understand the processes involved in the design and delivery of surveys and questionnaires, the principles of how questions are chosen and worded, and methods for answering the question selected are explored first. The chapter concludes by examining approaches to data presentation and analysis in quantitative research.

Choosing what questions to ask

The process of choosing what questions to ask within a quantitative research study requires planning. As a guiding principle, the nature of the study and the topic being explored will to some extent predetermine this. When deciding what questions to ask during a study it is important to keep in mind at all times the aims and objectives of the research.

One way in which the researcher can plan the questions to ask during a study is to examine the questions that other researchers have used in similar studies. However, while previous studies in similar areas can provide some general ideas, the exact nature of the research question and the characteristics of the people that the research is being undertaken with will be important in deciding which questions should be included in any study.

Many quantitative data collection tools already exist. Such tools, usually questionnaires, have been designed to collect defined data from within certain specific groups. Examples of these questionnaires include the Short Form 36 (SF36), which is a 36-question questionnaire that is used in general populations to gain an insight into individuals' perceptions of their own physical and psychological well-being. The SF36 is a useful tool for gaining data about the general well-being of individuals and has been used in many thousands of research projects (www.sf-36.org).

Disease-specific questionnaires have been especially designed to answer questions about the perceived state of health of individuals with a wide range of diseases. Examples include the 'Kidney Disease Quality of Life Short Form' (KDQOL – SF), used specifically with people with chronic kidney disease, and 'The MacNew Heart Disease Health-related Quality of Life Instrument', which is designed to assess and evaluate the health-related quality of life of people living with heart disease.

As well as questionnaires that apply to people in different health states, there are questionnaires for measuring physical well-being (e.g. Karnofsky Performance Scale Index), psychological well-being (e.g. Psychological General Well-being Index), social well-being (e.g. Social Activities Satisfaction Instrument) and emotional well-being (e.g. the State-Trait Anxiety Index). The benefit of using pre-existing questionnaires comes not only in the time that they save but also in the fact that (if matched appropriately) they often have a high degree of validity and reliability because they have been widely tested.

There is little point in designing questions for quantitative research when existing tools can address the study aims adequately. One note of caution should be given, however: just because a data collection instrument has been widely used and has good reliability and validity does not mean that it will retain those qualities in every group of individuals with whom it is used. For example, a questionnaire that is designed to measure the quality of life in individuals with renal disease may not apply very well to individuals with heart disease. So pre-existing questionnaires can only be used with certainty in people similar to those in whom the questionnaire has been validated.

Perhaps the most important aspect of the process of deciding which questions to ask is deciding which questions do not need to be included. For example, if you are researching the implementation of a pre-operative fasting regime for general surgery, questions about the gender, age and ethnicity of the people answering the questionnaire may not be important. If, however, you are concerned with the understanding of and adherence to pre-operative patient instructions, it may be relevant to the purposes of the study to gain some insight into whether gender, age and ethnicity have an effect on whether people have actually understood, or been able to comply with, the instructions given to them.

Wording questions for research

Questions must make sense to the person being asked them. This may seem quite obvious; however, a number of issues can arise in the wording of a question that can make it difficult to understand, let alone answer.

The use of words that have multiple or vague meanings can make a question difficult to answer. For example, when exploring the effects of back pain on individuals, a question such as 'Since you have had your back pain have you been able to go out a lot?' has multiple potential meanings:

- 'go out' may be taken to mean 'go out socially', 'go out shopping' or 'go out into the garden';
- 'a lot' may mean daily, weekly or monthly depending on what is normal for the individual.

Such questions also ignore what the person was able to do before they had back pain and what, therefore, is normal for them. It may be more appropriate to ask whether the person's level of activity has changed as a result of the back pain rather than pitching what is clearly an ambiguous question.

Using technical words or jargon in a questionnaire that is to be applied to the general public can mean that the questions are not understood. For example, in nursing we might use terms such as 'venepuncture' or 'taking bloods' to describe the process of taking a blood sample from a patient for subsequent analysis. These terms, while they may have a distinct and clear meaning to us, may confuse or potentially even frighten a lay person. Using technical language in a questionnaire applied to non-professionals assumes that they use the language in the same way that you do.

Activity 5.1 — *Critical thinking*

When you next take a handover, make a note of all of the abbreviations and technical language that is used. Consider how they might sound to a patient or a new student nurse.

As the answer is based on your own area of practice, there is no outline answer at the end of the chapter.

Avoiding asking more than one question within a question is also important. For example, a question with a yes/no answer such as 'Did you have any pain and nausea following your operation?' may gain a positive response in three situations: the respondent had pain, but no nausea; the respondent had nausea but no pain; and the respondent had both pain and nausea. Conversely, the absence of either one of the symptoms might get a negative response when in fact this is not true. Asking a question with a double meaning such as this and getting an inaccurate response means that the validity of the question is poor. That is to say, the question is not actually measuring what it sets out to measure.

As a general rule, therefore, questions should be short and precise, and refer to only one issue of interest.

The use of leading questions can also seriously affect the validity of a study. Leading questions are ones that seem to imply a specific response. Such responses may not truly represent the feelings of the respondents, and this will result in the introduction of bias into the study. This bias means that no confidence can be placed in the answer to a given question, and the question will have to be discarded.

Leading questions are of most concern when they are contained within studies that are evaluative. For example, if you are using a questionnaire to evaluate the use of patient-controlled analgesia (PCA), a question such as 'Do you think the fact that you managed your own pain control was better for you than having to wait for a nurse to bring an injection?' tends to point to two distinct reasons why the individual would be happier with PCA. The first is the phrase 'the fact that you managed'. This places the control of the pain firmly with the individual, who is then responsible if it does not work. The second reason is that it is made quite plain they would have had to wait for pain relief had they not been on PCA. That would not be a good thing, would it?

Activity 5.2   *Communication*

Try this for one day. Make a note of all the questions that you are asked. Identify which ones you understood completely and which you did not. Try to identify which questions tend to suggest an answer and which you feel free to answer as you see fit.

As the answer is based on your own area of practice, there is no outline answer at the end of the chapter.

Open and closed questions

Essentially, there are two distinct types of questions that can be contained within any study: open questions and closed questions. The choice of style of question to be used will depend on how much detail is required in the answers, the overall aim of the study and the background research that has gone into designing the study.

Open questions ask the respondent for their knowledge, attitude or feelings. They often begin with 'what', 'why' or 'how'. 'Tell me' or 'describe' may also be used to start open questions. Examples include:

- what is it like to survive cancer?
- why did you choose to be treated here?
- how was your stay in hospital?
- tell me what happened when you received your diagnosis.
- describe the clinic visit in more detail.

Open questions are problematic in quantitative research because they gain any number and variety of answers. The data obtained from these answers tend to contain more depth – assuming people can be bothered to answer them – and they allow the respondents to raise issues that are important to them. The variety and depth of the responses do mean, however, that it is almost impossible for researchers to quantify them in any meaningful way. The pros and cons of open questions are summarised in Table 5.1.

Table 5.1: Pros and cons of open questions

Pros	*Cons*
Provide rich in-depth data	Difficult to capture all answers
Do not restrict participants' answers	More difficult for participants to answer
Get more detailed answers	More difficult to categorise and analyse answers
Gain good insight into participant's opinions	May produce answers not relevant to the question
Let respondents raise issues	May allow people not to bother to answer questions fully

Closed questions are the exact opposite of open questions and are designed to get either a one word answer or a very short factual answer. They are very useful for quantitative data collection as the responses given are easily counted and analysed. They are quick and easy for respondents to answer. Because closed questions are quite focused, they tend towards directing people's answers. Examples include:

- do you feel lucky to have survived cancer?
- did you choose to be treated here because of our reputation?
- was your stay in hospital satisfactory?
- did you understand what you were told when you received your diagnosis?
- was your clinic visit okay?

The pros and cons of closed questions are summarised in Table 5.2.

Table 5.2: Pros and cons of closed questions

Pros	*Cons*
Quick to answer	Can be leading
Easy to understand	Respondents can only answer in ways the question allows
Engage people, including those with limited literacy skills	Respondents cannot raise new issues
Easy to quantify responses	
Avoid overly lengthy answers	

Because closed questions are designed to gain short responses, there are sometimes issues with their ability to fully capture the response that an individual wishes to give. This may mean that the findings of a quantitative study have limited validity because the answers gained are less than a true reflection of what the individual respondents wanted to say. This lack of **sensitivity** may be overcome by adapting the way in which closed questions can be responded to.

Scaling question responses

Scaling, or ranking, allows people involved in a study to choose an answer to a question that is closest in meaning to the answer they want to give. Such scales usually take one of three forms in quantitative studies: agreement, evaluation and frequency. It is usual for such scales to contain between four and seven options, with five being the most common. These methods of grouping responses are referred to as Likert items in some textbooks.

Agreement scales (see Figure 5.1) allow the respondent to match their level of agreement with a statement contained within a question. While agreement with the answers available may not be absolute, it is generally sufficient, within the context of the quantitative study, that the respondent is invited to choose the response that most closely fits what they think or feel.

| Strongly agree | Agree | Undecided | Disagree | Strongly disagree |

Figure 5.1: An example of an agreement scale

Evaluation scales (see Figure 5.2) allow for the respondent to answer in a manner that measures how good or bad they rated an experience, process or product. Because of the way they are worded, evaluation scales may encourage respondents to answer questions in a more honest way than an agreement scale, the questions for which can appear to be directive (leading).

| Excellent | Very good | Undecided | Poor | Very poor |

Figure 5.2: An example of an evaluation scale

Frequency scales (see Figure 5.3) allow the respondent to choose a response to a question that allows some idea as to whether the response represents their experience on all, some or only a very few occasions.

| Always | Usually | Sometimes | Rarely | Never |

Figure 5.3: An example of a frequency scale

What can be seen from the above three examples is that they invite a response to three slightly different questions: the first seeks agreement with a statement of fact; the second asks the respondent to rate an experience; and the third allows some feedback about whether the quality of an experience is consistently good.

Because each form of scaling gains a slightly different response, it is important that the researcher takes care during the design of the questions to refer back to the purpose of the study on a regular basis in order to maintain focus. In some instances it may be appropriate to have a mix of question styles in order to gain a more complete picture of the answers that the participants want to give.

Visual analogue scales

A visual analogue scale (VAS) (see Figure 5.4) provides another way of measuring responses to closed questions in a manner that increases their sensitivity. A VAS attempts to measure an attitude or feeling that spans a continuum of values and that cannot easily be precisely measured. In the clinical setting, the use of a VAS may help in understanding the amount of pain that a patient is suffering. Pain may range across a continuum from no pain through to severe pain, and the range in a VAS is continuous to reflect this. Pain does not take discrete leaps, as the use of an agreement, evaluation or frequency scale might seem to suggest. A VAS is another example of a Likert scale.

Certainly, the level of accuracy that such a scale allows is more than is necessary in most quantitative studies. However, the advantages of the VAS in engaging people with limited literacy skills and in applying measures to variables that are difficult to quantify makes the VAS a useful research tool.

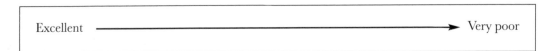

Figure 5.4: An example of a visual analogue scale

By convention, the line used in a VAS is 10 cm long. Because of their highly subjective nature, VASs are not easy to use to compare the scores given between individuals, but they have great benefits when trying to quantify the changes in feeling, e.g. the amount of pain, of an individual. These scales have the disadvantage that the response needs to be measured in order to be quantifiable, so more time is needed to collect the data required.

In children, or adults with very limited literacy skills, the use of pictures instead of a written-on single-line scale can enhance the ability of the researcher to collect data. Perhaps the best example is the use of the 'faces pain scale' which rates the pain that a child is feeling by relating it to the emotion displayed on cartoon faces (Spagrud et al., 2003) (e.g. see www.wongbaker faces.org).

Surveys

Key features

Surveys fall broadly into the research methodology that was identified in Chapter 4 as cross-sectional. That is, they attempt to quantify the prevalence of a variable (e.g. feeling, attitude or opinion) in a group of individuals at a given point in time. Surveys set out to be either descriptive or correlational. A descriptive study only presents single variables in the amount that they occur within the study sample, while a correlational study looks for associations between two or more variables (e.g. whether age correlates with satisfaction with hospital care).

While a survey may be able to demonstrate an apparent correlation between two variables, because it is not longitudinal (it does not carry through time) it is not a method that can prove a cause-and-effect relationship. (To remind yourself about this distinction, see Chapter 4.)

Broadly speaking, surveys can be undertaken prospectively (that is in real time), retrospectively (that is, using previously collected data) or using a mixture of both approaches.

Prospective surveys

Prospective surveys are undertaken to ascertain the feelings, thoughts and attitudes of people about a service or product at the point at which they receive the service or use the product. This has the advantage that the data collected can all be standardised, ensuring their reliability. That is, the ways in which the data is collected are managed by the researcher, and are therefore not subject to individual idiosyncrasies.

Prospective data collection has the added advantage that it does not require the person to have to remember a previous event; they can record feelings etc. in real time. This means that recall bias is eliminated from the study.

Retrospective surveys

Retrospective surveys are studies that collect data about past events. Some surveys may use previously collected data – for example, routinely recorded data on outpatient waiting times – or they may collect data from individuals about a service or product that they experienced in the past.

In common with all retrospective studies, retrospective surveys are prone to issues that relate to the ability of an individual to recall past events (recall bias); clearly, time can change a person's perceptions and memories of an event. Retrospective surveys using previously collected data are also subject to the quality of the data collection processes at the time. There may be issues with reliability and possibly validity because data were not collected according to a standardised format and the consistency of the data may be questionable.

> **Concept summary: recall bias**
>
> Recall bias can prove a major obstacle in the execution of any study. It arises in a number of ways, all of which are systematic. People who had a bad experience of care may be more likely to remember it as being bad than people who had a reasonable experience, who may, with the passing of time, subsequently remember the experience as being good. Mothers of children with birth defects are more likely to recall the use of alcohol and smoking during pregnancy than mothers whose children are born healthy.

The quality and consistency of data collection and recording outside a research project are variable. For example, the notes recorded by two triage nurses working in the same emergency department may be quite different, even if they are seeing people with similar conditions. This is a result of normal human variation, but it means that the collection of data for research purposes may be incomplete. Even within research there need to be safeguards in place, especially where more than one person is collecting data, to make sure there is some consistency.

Advantages

Surveys have the advantage of being quick and easy to do, and this makes them relatively cheap. Because surveys are so commonplace in society they are easily understood by people, and therefore generally quite user friendly.

Surveys can be undertaken using a variety of different approaches, which include the use of questionnaires (which may be postal or administered via face-to-face interviews, telephone interviews, e-mail, online chat rooms or dedicated websites). The variety of techniques available to undertake a survey means that there has to be a degree of thought applied to how a survey is to be undertaken, with some topic areas more suitable for a particular method than others.

On the whole, face-to-face interviews yield the fullest responses with the highest uptake of respondents. This is because it is harder to refuse a face-to-face interview than it is to ignore an e-mail and because there is the opportunity in a face-to-face interview for the questioner to clarify any questions that the respondent does not understand, as well as to clarify any responses.

Disadvantages

Because of their speed and the fact that they need to be user friendly, surveys tend to be somewhat superficial. Furthermore, the quality of the data collected in a survey is limited by the willingness and ability of the individuals included in the study to answer the questions posed to them. The willingness of participants to answer the questions is related to the topic of the research, the questions that are being asked, and how the questions are being asked.

When not filled in face to face, surveys may be responded to by people other than those they were sent to – this can potentially bias the study as it affects the sample selection. Mailed and e-mailed surveys are easily ignored, and if they can be returned anonymously, it is hard to chase up recipients.

People who respond to surveys are self-selecting, that is, they choose to take part. This self-selection may result in bias, with individuals with a very good or very bad experience being more likely to take part, for instance, than people having an average, or normal experience.

Structured interviews

Structured interviews are interviews in which the questions to be asked and the order in which they are to be asked are decided before the interview takes place. The interviewer has a list of the questions they want to ask and then asks them. There is no room allowed for deviation from the interview script, which has to be delivered in the same order using the same words on each occasion it is used (Tod, 2006).

Structured interviews have the advantage that all of the interviewees are questioned in the same way, following the same protocol. This makes the job of the interviewer that little bit easier. It allows there to be some consistency within a research process that involves one researcher but also in studies that involve more than one person in the data collection.

Concept summary: structured interviews

Structured interviews are in some respects similar to the documents used when undertaking an assessment of a patient on admission to a ward. It is important that all of the same data are collected in the same manner so that everyone who is later involved in the patient's care has access to the data in a structured and consistent manner. Deviating from the assessment process, neglecting to collect some pieces of information, or failing to include all of the usual documentation in the assessment leads to confusion and the potential for something important to be missed. Within the structured interview protocol, failure to gather data in the same way on each occasion means the data will not easily be compared and that there is confusion about what questions the research has actually answered.

It is easier when writing up a study involving structured interviews to include in the research paper the list of questions asked and the order in which they were asked. This has the advantage of making it clear to readers exactly what was asked, so they can then compare this to the answers given and decide for themselves if the findings of the study, as presented by the researcher, appear reasonable.

The main disadvantage of structured interviews is that they tend to gain less full responses from the interviewees, as the answers they can give are constrained by the type and nature of the questions asked. Structured interviews are sometimes used as a method of data collection in quantitative research where there is a requirement for all of the data to be collected in the same way using the same questions in order to maintain the consistency (reliability) of the data collection.

Activity 5.3	*Critical thinking*

When you next work clinically, pay attention to the way in which people answer the questions you pose to them. Pay special attention to the length and quality of the answers given when you are collecting very well-structured data (as you might on admission, or when preparing someone for surgery). Compare the quality (what we have identified as depth and richness) of the answers you get from people when you ask them more unstructured questions when interacting with them on a more social level, perhaps at mealtimes or when doing clinical observations.

As this answer is based on your observations, there is no outline answer at the end of the chapter.

Questionnaires

As a method of data collection questionnaires are everywhere. There are many different styles of questionnaire, each designed to do a different job. Some questionnaires are specially written for an individual piece of research, while others have been designed to be used time and again to measure variables within defined populations.

Questionnaires can be delivered in a number of ways, which include face to face, via post, via e-mail and online.

There are advantages and disadvantages to all of the different types and delivering methods. The nature of the research and the research question itself guide the exact choice of how a questionnaire is both designed and delivered. There are few hard-and-fast rules about what a good questionnaire should contain in the way of questions or ways of answering. Nor are there any guiding principles that allow the researcher to know which method of delivering the questionnaire is most appropriate for the research question they are investigating.

What is important in the choice of style of questions and mode of delivery of the questionnaire is that the researcher has thought about the potential pros and cons, given the nature of the research question and the people to whom the questionnaire is to be applied. The best researcher will refer, as we have seen in Chapter 1, to the existing literature in the topic area and use the lessons learnt from this to guide their decisions. For the novice researcher this is particularly important, as is the engagement of the help of a more experienced researcher and potentially a statistician who can advise on question designs that will support the subsequent process of data analysis.

Key features

For the quantitative questionnaire, the thing that is most important is that the answers collected are a true reflection of the question asked. This may seem quite obvious; however, writing a question in such a way that it will be understood to mean the same thing by all the people who will read it is not all that easy.

The second most important aspect of questionnaire design is to ensure that responses are gained from as many of the target sample as possible. This means that thought needs to go into not only the questions asked but also where, when and how the questioning is to take place. In a student or young population, a questionnaire may work well when placed in an online environment, but the opposite may be true for older people or those on low incomes who may not have access to, or be used to using the internet.

Questionnaires often need to elicit more than one type of data. The main data relate to the topic of interest while other data are needed to record the demographic and other characteristics of respondents. The length of any questionnaire should be limited to gaining the data needed for the study and no more. It is often wise to include some filtering questions at the start so that people not eligible for the study are identified early on.

Generally, it is a good idea to phrase questions positively rather than negatively, for example, using 'Was your pain well managed after surgery?' as opposed to 'Was your pain poorly controlled after surgery?' The use of negative questioning can, however, be used to check two things. First, when asking for an opinion about something, asking the same question later on in the questionnaire but in the opposite way can be used to check the consistency of an individual's answers – so if they answer 'disagree' to the ranking of a positive question, they should answer 'agree' to the ranking of a negative question. Second, it is possible to see if the respondent is actually reading all of the questions rather than assuming their content. If they are assuming the content and the question format varies, this is likely to result in a few questions to which the answers do not correspond.

Other ways of checking the quality of the questioning process include the use of open questions that allow the respondent to record their own response and comparing these to the closed responses. Repeat measures designs allow the researcher to apply the questionnaire to the same person at different points in time to see if there is consistency. Of course, this type of design is onerous and relies on a respondent being willing to fill out the same questionnaire twice. The disadvantage of this approach arises when the research relates to thoughts, feelings and opinions that are subject to change over time anyway.

Questionnaires do not write themselves and there are a number of routes to checking the quality of a questionnaire you have written yourself. Using experts in the topic being studied to help write the questions can be fruitful as they often know the sorts of ideas and misconceptions that people have. Doing a pilot study of the questionnaire using the sort of people who will be involved in the main study is also a useful way of ensuring the questions make sense and filling in the questionnaire is not too onerous.

The length of a questionnaire will impact on the response rates achieved. A shorter tick-box questionnaire will always gain more responses than long, more complex ones. It would be wrong to think that a long questionnaire is necessarily of better quality than a short one that is better focused.

The order in which questions appear has an impact on whether or not people decide to fill in a questionnaire, as do the quality and nature of the questioning involved. Once people have committed some time to filling in a questionnaire they are more likely to finish it. The general rules for sequencing questions are summarised below.

> **Concept summary: rules about sequencing questions**
>
> - Go from general to specific.
> - Go from easy to harder.
> - Go from factual to more abstract.
> - Start with closed format questions (scaled).
> - Start with questions about the main subject.
> - Don't start with personal or demographic questions.

Administering questionnaires

There are many ways of administering a questionnaire. The choice of delivery will tend to be driven by the nature of the questions and the sample being questioned. Self-administered questionnaires may be posted in the mail, be placed online (perhaps in a topical chat room), be e-mailed or be left in a pertinent clinical area, perhaps. Interviewer-administered questionnaires may be undertaken face to face, over the telephone or even via the internet.

There are a number of pros and cons of each approach, and these need to be considered before launching into the questioning process. Table 5.3 summarises the pros of each approach.

Table 5.3: Pros of self- and interviewer-administered questionnaires

Self-administered questionnaires	*Interviewer-administered questionnaires*
Quick, cheap, easy to administer, convenient to respondent, confidentiality and anonymity easily preserved, easily standardised format and limited researcher input needed.	Interviewer can clarify questions, allows participation by people who are illiterate, virtually guarantees a high response rate, quality and completeness of questionnaires may be higher.

Presenting and analysing quantitative data

By their very nature quantitative studies produce outputs – findings – that are quantifiable. This means that the findings of a quantitative study include data that use numbers. The presentation of data from a quantitative study includes data that describe both the characteristics of the participants and the findings of the study. As well as the descriptive data, statistics may be presented that make inferences about what the study has found. These two types of statistical data are called **descriptive statistics** and **inferential statistics**.

Essentially, descriptive statistics describe only the range, frequency and distribution of certain characteristics within the study. Inferential statistics, on the other hand, present data about the probabilities associated with the outcomes of the study. The following sections discuss in limited detail the sort of data that should be included in the report of a quantitative research study and why. Some explanation of how different statistical findings are arrived at is offered. You are encouraged to look in the specialist texts suggested at the end of the chapter if you want to be able to understand any of the information presented here in more detail or if you need to undertake any statistical tests for your own research.

Descriptive statistics

Descriptive statistics do exactly what they say. That is, they describe patterns of data within a data set. Descriptive statistics are used to give the reader some idea of the make-up of a study, the numbers of people involved, their spread of age, gender, ethnicity and the like. The exact data to be presented depend on the nature and purpose of the study undertaken and will therefore vary.

Descriptive statistics are concerned with the presentation of summaries of the data generated during a study. Examples of the ways in which descriptive statistics are presented include basic calculations, graphs, charts and tables. Descriptive statistics present an account of the data, with particular reference to its central tendency, distribution and frequency.

Measures of central tendency

Measures of central tendency give the reader a good idea of some of the central, or average, values of a set of data. There are a number of measures of central tendency, each with particular messages that they convey to the reader of the study. They also allow the researcher to make some statements about the nature of the sample from which the data were collected and the overall results of the study.

The arithmetic mean

This is what is commonly known as an **average**. The **mean** is calculated by adding all of the values in a data set together and then dividing by the number of values. For example, all the ages of the people involved in the study divided by the number of people involved in the study would give us the mean age (see Figure 5.5).

The mean uses all the observations in the data set and each observation affects the mean. It is sensitive to extreme values (i.e. extremely large or small data can cause the mean to be pulled toward the extreme data). The mean has valuable mathematical properties that make it convenient for use in inferential statistical analysis too, as we will see later in the chapter.

Find the arithmetic mean of the data: 7, 5, 4, 6, 7, 14, 11, 5, 9, 10, 12

$7 + 5 + 4 + 6 + 7 + 14 + 11 + 5 + 9 + 10 + 12 = 90$

$90 \div 11 = 8.2$

Figure 5.5: An example of how to calculate a mean

The median

The **median** is the middle value in an *ordered* set of values (see Figure 5.6). If there is an even number of data in the set, the median is the mean of the two middle numbers. The median provides a better measure of central tendency, on the whole, than the mean when there are some extremely large or small observations in a data set.

Unlike the mean, the median does not have important mathematical properties for use in future calculations. The median is often used when quoting survival data in the clinical setting and refers to the point in time to which 50 per cent of patients with a given condition will be expected to survive.

Find the median of the data:	7, 5, 4, 6, 7, 14, 11, 5, 9, 10, 12
Put the data in order:	4, 5, 5, 6, 7, 7, 9, 10, 11, 12, 14
Select the middle value:	4, 5, 5, 6, 7, 7, 9, 10, 11, 12, 14 = 7

Figure 5.6: An example of how to calculate a median

The mode

The **mode** is the most frequently occurring number in a set of observations. Some data sets may have two modes, in which case we say the data are *bimodal* (see Figure 5.7). Where a data set has more than two modes it is referred to as *multimodal*. The mode is not usually a helpful measure of central tendency because there can be more than one mode or even no mode. Like the median, the mode does not have important mathematical properties for future use.

The mode might be useful in reporting people's attitudes or opinions, especially when the data collected are nominal or categorical.

Find the mode of the data:	7, 5, 4, 6, 7, 14, 11, 5, 9, 10, 12

The numbers 5 and 7 both appear twice; each other number appears only once.
The dataset is therefore bimodal with the numbers 5 and 7 both being the modes of this dataset.

Figure 5.7: An example of how to calculate a mode

The range

The **range** is the difference between the largest observation of a data set and the smallest observation. Typically the smallest and largest number, e.g. the age of the youngest and oldest people in a study, are reported.

The major disadvantage of the range is that it does not include all of the observations. Only the two most extreme values are included and these two numbers may be untypical observations.

Using the same data as Figure 5.7, therefore, the range of the observations is from 4 to 14 and is therefore 10.

Standard deviation

This is perhaps the most poorly understood of the descriptive statistics reported in any study. Standard deviation is essentially the mean of the difference from the mean of each of the observations being reported. The best way to understand standard deviation is perhaps to see one worked out long hand – see Figure 5.8.

---

1. Find the arithmetic mean of the data: 7, 5, 4, 6, 7, 14, 11, 5, 9, 10, 12 = 8.2

2. Find the difference between each observation and the mean (e.g. 7 – 8.2= *–1.2*).
    –1.2, –3.2, –4.2, –2.2, –1.2, 5.8, 2.8, –3.2, 0.8, 1.8, 3.8

3. Square these differences (for example -1.2 x -1.2 = *1.44*).
    1.44+10.24+17.64+4.84+1.44+33.64+7.84+10.24+0.64+3.24+14.44

4. Add together these squared differences = 105.64

5. Divide this number by the number of observations minus one = 9.6.

6. Find the square root of this number = **3.1**

Figure 5.8: An example of how to calculate a standard deviation

The standard deviation of a set of data that are normally distributed (that is, data that when graphed show a bell shape) – as is the case in much biological data – enables the reader to get a feel for where most of the variables within a data set lie. Something in the region of 66 per cent of all the data will lie within one standard deviation of the mean, while 95 per cent of observations will lie within two standard deviations. The reporting of the mean and the standard deviation of a given data set allows the researcher and subsequent readers of the research to get a good feel for where most of the values within the data set lie.

It is a great relief to know that it is usually not necessary for the researcher to have to calculate these descriptive statistics manually, as all spreadsheet programmes now have this facility.

Activity 5.4   *Research and finding out*

Collect together the heights and weights of a few of your classmates or the people in your house. Using the definitions and examples above, calculate the mean, median, mode, standard deviation and range of this data.

As the answer is based on your own data, there is no outline answer at the end of the chapter.

Inferential statistics

Descriptive statistics are used to reduce down a data set of numbers into a few uncomplicated values that are represented either as numbers or in graphs. In this sense, descriptive statistics are like a book summary – they get across the basic idea without the detail.

The purpose of inferential statistics within the research process is to demonstrate that the findings of the research extend beyond the sample within which the research was carried out. Extending beyond the study sample to the population from which the sample was drawn requires that inferential statistics go beyond the data available as a result of the study. As a result of the fact that inferential statistics go beyond the actual data available via the study, they are invariably subject to error. Because of this potential for error the term 'inferential statistics' and not 'deductive statistics' is used.

> **Concept summary: inferential statistics**
>
> Inferential is a word used to indicate that the statistical findings are subject to some presumption on the part of the person doing the statistics. This presumptiveness is reflected in two ways: first, the findings of the inferential statistics are usually presented as probabilities (p values), which are explained below); second, the findings of all quantitative studies remain open to be proved or disproved by subsequent studies (as was discussed in Chapter 4).

Inferential statistics use a number of processes to make sure that the suppositions are as reasonable as they can be. What this means is that despite the fact that the findings are not 100 per cent certain, we can place a fair degree of confidence in the statistical findings of any quantitative research.

The findings of inferential statistics are usually expressed in terms of probability. The probability to which they refer is the chance of the findings of the study being found by chance. In other words, probability shows us how much confidence we can have that the findings of the study did not occur by fluke.

Probabilities are expressed as p values. For example, a p value of 0.1 (usually written up as p=0.1) would mean that there is a 10 per cent chance that the findings of the study occurred by chance. Think about how this works: 0.1 is one tenth of the number one, while 10 per cent is one tenth of 100 percent, so they are essentially the same thing.

Activity 5.5   *Research and finding out*

If p=0.1 means a 10 per cent chance or 1/10th chance that the findings of the study occurred by chance, try to work out what the following mean:

p=0.2
p=0.05

continued . . .

p=0.01

p=0.001

Express your answers as a percentage and as a non-decimal fraction.

There are answers at the end of the chapter.

In order to understand p values better, it is important to understand that the lower the number the better the result. For example, p=0.02 suggests that the findings of the study occurring by chance are four times less than if the result were p=0.08. Sometimes statistics are presented using less than ($<$) and greater than ($>$) symbols. Given that the smaller the number the less chance there is that the result of the study occurred by chance, clearly the best results will generally be small and the $<$ is preferable. So a result of $p<0.05$ means there is less than a one in 20 chance that the results of the study occurred by chance.

By convention, if there is no good statistical reason, a result of $p<0.05$ (probability of less than, or equal to ($\leq$) one in 20, is accepted as a statistically significant result. Statistically significant means that it is accepted that the results of the study did not occur by chance, or that at the very least the chance of them occurring by chance is so small as to be insignificant. Sometimes in sociological studies a p value of <0.1 is accepted as statistically significant as the burden of proof in this type of study is less than in quantitative studies.

Statistical significance is not the same as clinical significance. Some studies that demonstrate a weak statistical finding may well be important, or significant, enough for clinicians to consider adopting the findings. The most important reason for this is the fact that some studies have small sample sizes, which can seriously affect the statistics. Weak statistical significance in small studies tends to suggest that the study might have reached a more statistically significant result had it been bigger, and for many clinical purposes this may be enough on which to base a tentative change.

Before looking briefly at some of the inferential statistical tests that can be used in analysing quantitative research data, it is perhaps worth understanding the different types of data that can be analysed.

Data types

During the collection of data for any study there are a number of ways in which the data can be categorised (see Table 5.4). Categorising the data helps in the selection of both the descriptive and the inferential statistics to be applied to the data and is something that should be thought about and designed into the study at the start in order to ensure that the correct data are collected in the correct manner to allow later presentation or analysis.

Different data types can be presented in different ways using descriptive statistics. Table 5.5 shows the measures of central tendency (types of average) that can be used to describe different data types.

Table 5.4: Types of quantitative data

Data type	Type of measurement	Example
Categorical	Nominal (has no inherent order)	Diagnosis; ethnicity
	Ordinal (categories with an order)	A Likert scale; Self-reported health status
	Binary (a form of ordinal involving only two groups)	Gender; illness or wellness
Quantitative (interval or ratio) (units of measurement applied as a rule)	Discrete (as a rule these are whole numbers)	Number of patients on a ward; blood group
	Continuous (can take any value, but usually measured, counted or ordered to a predetermined degree of accuracy)	Height; weight; temperature

Table 5.5: Measures of central tendency that can be used with specific quantitative data types

	Type of average		
	Mean	Median	Mode
Nominal			X
Ordinal		X	X
Interval/ratio	X	X	X

Parametric/non-parametric data

Before applying any inferential statistics to a data set it is important to ascertain whether the data need to be analysed using parametric or non-parametric statistical tests. Parametric data are data that when plotted on a histogram present a bell-shaped curve. Such data are said to be normally distributed (Altman, 1991). Normal distribution is most often achieved in data sets that are large and that contain naturally occurring measurements (such as heights of a group).

Data that are normally distributed (i.e. produce a bell-shaped curve) have at their peak the mean of the data with about 68 per cent of the data values lying within one standard deviation of the mean, 95 per cent within two and 99.7 per cent within three (see Figure 5.9). As well as plotting the distribution curve, there are statistical tests that can be applied to data to see if they are normally distributed and therefore whether parametric tests can be used in the analysis of the data.

Parametric tests tend to be the preferred form of statistical testing because they produce more powerful results on the whole. However, the incorrect use of parametric tests in small data sets, or with data that are not normally distributed, can lead to misleading results.

The exact choice of test to be used with different forms of data is a matter of careful consideration that is best decided before data for a study are collected, and this is best decided in

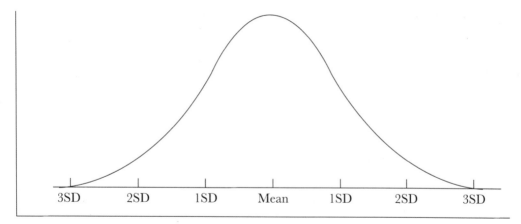

Figure 5.9: The normal distribution curve

conjunction with a statistician. Given the variety and number of statistical tests available, it is beyond the scope of this book to present these here. Instead we will consider the use and interpretation of two commonly used statistical tests that will allow us to get some insight into how inferential statistics work.

The t-test

The first common inferential statistic is the *t-test*. The t-test is used to gauge whether the means of two groups are statistically different from each other. Not only this, the t-test is sensitive to the spread of the individual results within each group (as represented by the standard deviation; see page 105) and the number of observations in each set of data.

The t-test comes in two forms: the standard t-test compares the means from two separate (independent) groups (as one might find in a randomised controlled trial where there is an experimental group and a control group) and the paired t-test measures before and after measurements in the same individual (where an intervention has applied, for example) or in two paired (or matched, such as for gender, age and ethnicity) individuals.

The standard t-test can only be applied to data that are continuous (see Table 5.4) and that follow the normal distribution (see Figure 5.9) and where the two groups' standard deviations (see Figure 5.8) are broadly similar.

> ## Case study
>
> *In the study by Isoyama et al. (2012) (cited in Chapter 4, page 73) the standard t-test was used at the start of the study to ensure the two groups enrolled were broadly similar for certain characteristics (in this case age and years of infertility treatment) at the start of the study. The null hypothesis is that the groups are different in some important respect. The calculated probabilities (p values) are 1 and 0.1351, which means the null hypothesis is not proven (remember p must be 0.05 or less for this to be the case).*

continued . . .

> *It is useful to note that demonstrating the similarity of the groups at the start of the study is important in showing that the findings of the study are due to the intervention and not some other difference between the groups that occurred at randomisation.*

The paired t-test has slightly different rules in that they apply to the set of difference scores; the observations should be normally distributed (for both readings); the readings should be paired and in preference the dependent variable will be measured on an interval or ratio scale.

Three applications of the paired t-test that are useful but slightly different are: to compare the efficacy of two forms of eye drops for hay fever relief when drop A is applied to the right eye and drop B to the left eye in the same individual (this gives a binary result (relief or no relief)) where the individual is their own 'pair'; to measure the impact of an exercise regime over a one-month period in people weighed at the start and the end of the exercise programme (continuous data) where again the individual is their own pair; and to measure the growth rate in twins where one is given a supplement and the other a normal diet (here the pairing is closely matched).

The chi-square test

The other important statistical test widely used in quantitative research is the *chi-square (X^2) test*. The chi-square test can be applied to data that: report frequency (categorical data); are of an adequate size; and where the categories being used are mutually exclusive (that is, no one subject can be in any two groups at the same time). The chi-square test basically allows us to see if the distributions (counts) of categorical data differ between one or more groups. It is worth noting that the chi-square test can only be used on actual numbers and not percentages, proportions or means.

Case study

In their cross-sectional study of the association between smoking and the bipolar affective disorder and smoking, Kreinin et al. (2012) demonstrated a statistically significant association between smoking and alcohol abuse as well as between smoking and the use of non-alcoholic psychoactive agents using the chi-square test (cited in Chapter 4, page 85).

You may find it useful to look up the studies cited here to look at how the statistical data are presented. Alternatively, look up some other research papers and review how they present their descriptive and inferential statistics.

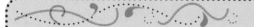

Chapter summary

This chapter has introduced you to the key methods used in data collection in the types of quantitative research that nurses most frequently undertake, that is, questionnaires and surveys. Such methods are often used to answer questions about the perceptions and attitudes of participants to the care they have received.

We have established that the validity and reliability of the data collected are affected by the ways in which questions are worded and presented. Validity, which is about ensuring that a research tool measures what it sets out to measure, is affected by the choice of questions used, while reliability is ensured when the data have been collected in a way that is readily reproducible.

We have seen that there are a variety of ways that both surveys and questionnaires can be undertaken and that the choice of approach is affected by the type of question being asked. Sometimes the nature of the questions asked requires sensitive face-to-face delivery, while on other occasions the sheer volume that can be achieved by a self-completion questionnaire enables a study to attain a high degree of statistical significance.

We have seen how to present and analyse the data from a quantitative study and that decisions about how to analyse and present data need to be made before data collection has started. We have seen that numerical data can be dealt with in two ways, descriptive statistics – which merely describe the data – and inferential statistics – which make inferences about the data that go beyond the data collected. Making inferences about the data that go beyond the sample mean that the findings of the study become more generalisable, with the likelihood of the finding being a result of chance being represented by the p value calculated.

Activities: Brief outline answers

Activity 5.5: Research and finding out (pages 106–7)

p=0.2 means 20% or 1/5th chance
p=0.05 means 5% or 1/20th chance
p=0.01 means: 1% or 1/100th chance
p=0.001 means: 0.1% or 1/1000th chance

Further reading

McKenna, H, Hasson, F and Keeney, S (2006) Surveys, in Gerish, K and Lacey, A (eds) *The research process in nursing* (5th edn). Oxford: Blackwell.

A good discussion of various survey methods.

Meadows, KA (2003) So you want to do research? 5: questionnaire design. *British Journal of Community Nursing.* 8 (12): 562–70.

An overview of questionnaire design.

Plichta, SB and Kelvin, E (eds) (2013) *Munro's Statistical Methods for Health Care Research*, 6th edition. London: Wolters Kluwer/Lippincott Williams and Wilkins.

A very clear and comprehensive book covering major statistical methods.

Polit, DF and Beck CT (2008) *Nursing research: generating and assessing evidence for nursing practice* (8th edn). London: Wolters Kluwer/Lippincott Williams & Wilkins.

Part Five (Analyzing and interpreting research data) provides a high-quality discussion of data analysis.

Useful websites

http://mste.illinois.edu/hill/dstat/dstat.html A rather wacky but informative introduction to descriptive statistics.

www.rlo-cetl.ac.uk:8080/open_virtual_file_path/i281n6662t/design/index.html Website outlining good practice in questionnaire design.

www.socialresearchmethods.net/kb/statdesc.php A concise but useful introduction to descriptive statistics.

www.socialresearchmethods.net/kb/analysis.php Some very useful information about descriptive and inferential statistics.

www.socialresearchmethods.net/kb/statinf.php A very helpful guide to inferential statistics.

www.statpac.com/surveys/ A useful tutorial on survey and questionnaire design.

www.wongbakerfaces.org Look here to see one example of a visual analogue 'faces pain scale'.

companion website

For further activities and other useful material, visit the companion website at
www.sagepub.co.uk/ellis_research2e

Chapter 6
Multiple methods, evaluation and action research

NMC Standards for Pre-registration Nursing Education

This chapter will address the following competencies:

Domain 1: Professional values

4. All nurses must work in partnership with service users, carers, families, groups, communities and organisations. They must manage risk, and promote health and wellbeing while aiming to empower choices that promote self-care and safety.

Domain 4: Leadership, management and team working

2. All nurses must systematically evaluate care and ensure that they and others use the findings to help improve people's experience and care outcomes and to shape future services.

NMC Essential Skills Clusters

This chapter will address the following ESCs:

Care, compassion and communication

1. As partners in the care process, people can trust a newly registered graduate nurse to provide collaborative care based on the highest standards, knowledge and competence

For entry to the register:

12. Recognises and acts to overcome barriers in developing effective relationships with service users and carers.

Chapter aims

After reading this chapter, you will be able to:

*   identify the major features of evaluation and action research;
*   describe the advantages and disadvantages of triangulation of data collection methodologies;
*   describe the purpose of research in and on action;
*   demonstrate awareness of the purpose of action orientated research in nursing practice.

Introduction

So far in this book we have seen that research methodologies are split between those that are qualitative and those that are quantitative. We have explored some of the methods used within these methodologies and how they might be analysed. In this chapter we will explore the idea that some approaches to research use both methods in order to answer questions about practice.

It is important at this stage to recognise that research in nursing (and in health and social care in general) is about the application of research to practice in order to change it for the better. Nursing is all about action – that is, doing things for, and perhaps more importantly with, patients in order to improve their lives. It is beyond the scope of this book to explore this idea in any detail, but the concepts of using evidence – of which research is only one element – to inform and improve nursing practice are explored in some detail in *Evidenced-based Practice in Nursing* in this series.

In this chapter, we examine the concepts that underpin the use of triangulated research methods, evaluation research and action research. The purpose of this exploration is to broaden the understanding of approaches to research in health and social care, and what they can be used to achieve.

The key features of the research approaches discussed in this chapter are that they are focused very much on the practice of nursing and not on the generation of ideas for later application. That is to say, the processes involved in evaluation and action research are focused on solving clinical and practice issues in real time. In this respect they differ greatly from the methodologies described elsewhere in the book, which have focused on the generation of knowledge leading to the need for further research and/or the need for the generation of strategies and policies for the adoption of the findings of the research into clinical practice.

The use of a single methodology in research has been described as *methodological separatism* (Henderson, 1993). Methodological separatism arises out of the fact that various researchers within different disciplines believe the human world can only be studied in ways that are distinct and separate from the non-human world. For example, we can study the healing of a broken bone using radiographic and scientific techniques (non-human), but to understand what it is like to experience the healing of a broken bone it is necessary to ask someone who has experienced it first-hand what it is like (human). It is not a debate so much about whether qualitative or quantitative research is more legitimate or better. Rather, this separatist view of the world regards humanity and the study of humanity as being something completely separate from everything else.

This separatist view is perhaps too simplistic for the meaningful study of humans, healthcare and nursing in that it fails to recognise the interconnectedness of human biology, sociology, psychology and philosophy. We are all aware, as nurses, that the activities of daily living are interconnected. The biological reality of pain affects the psychological well-being of our patients. Psychological distress impacts on their social well-being. Their social well-being impacts on the way in which they view the world. The way in which we view the world impacts on the way in which we experience pain, and so the cycle goes on.

Research in nursing involves research into people, and methodological separatism fails to recognise the complexity of human beings and the ways in which our social and biological beings are inextricably linked.

The exploration of triangulation of research methods is intended to demonstrate that healthcare problems are complex and the solutions to them are therefore quite complex and multifaceted. That is to say, high quality healthcare, and nursing care in particular, is about more than the mere management or curing of disease and as much about the experience of the care from the point of view of the patient. To this end, the triangulation of research methods allows the exploration of both the quantitative and the qualitative elements of care.

Triangulation

As we have seen in the book so far, the different research methodologies and associated methods each have different advantages and disadvantages. Given each methodology and method has its weaknesses, it makes some sense for researchers to employ a variety of approaches within their research in order to minimise the impact of these failings.

For example, the weaknesses that might be associated with the narrative data collection methods include that people can tell the researcher whatever they want to say, and the researcher has no way of knowing if what they say is, in fact, true. The weakness of an observation might be that the observer sees only what someone is doing and how they are doing it, without understanding why they are acting in that manner. Taken together, therefore, observation and interviews (as often seen in ethnographic participant observation) can act in a complementary manner, allowing the subject of the research both to demonstrate they act in a certain way and to explain what motivates them to act in that way. The collection of data using two or more methods therefore gives a more rounded, or complete, picture of the activity someone is undertaking. The data collected by these methods are sometimes described as being richer or deeper than the data collected by the use of one method alone. There are also times, however, when the data collected may appear contradictory, and significant discernment is needed on the part of the researchers to understand why this might have occurred, and how it might be overcome in the analysis and explanation of the findings.

As well as collecting data in more than one way (for example, using qualitative and quantitative techniques), triangulation in research can be achieved by two or more researchers collecting data on the same phenomenon using the same, or broadly similar, methods. This technique might be useful in observational research – for example, where there may be differences, or discrepancies, in what people notice in the same or similar situations. As such, this methodological triangulation of data collection allows the researcher to test the reliability and validity of the data they are collecting.

Activity 6.1   *Communication*

The purpose of triangulation is to improve upon perspective, to understand an issue from more than one view and to therefore gain insights that may not be readily available if only one approach to the research is used. To understand this, think about what it means to you as a nurse to provide care for an identified patient recovering from surgery or on the ward with a medical condition.

continued . . .

As nurses, we see the biological, physical and some aspects of the emotional response of the individual to what has happened to them. Now spend some time talking to the same patient about what it means to them to be in the hospital and what the experience they have had is like. What you may notice is that they will have a particular perspective on what has happened and while this perspective will in some ways be similar to the one you have, there will be subtle, but very distinct differences.

As the answer is based on your own observations, there is no outline answer at the end of the chapter.

Triangulation of research methods also has the potential effect of reducing the amount of **bias** within a study. Bias can arise out of the ways in which data are collected (for example, power imbalances within a focus group can lead to the views of the most powerful becoming more dominant). Such **measurement biases** can be overcome if more than one method of collecting the data is used (for example, a questionnaire or survey being applied as well). Other forms of bias include **response bias** when an individual answers in a manner that they believe that the researcher wants them to (the Hawthorne effect). The collection of data in another manner, perhaps anonymously, may help overcome such problems.

Sampling bias is another frequent problem in studies that seek to gain insights into the understandings or beliefs of large populations. The use of a single method of data collection such as online surveys may exclude people who do not have access to the internet. Triangulating data collection methods by also undertaking face-to-face interviews in the street may serve to decrease sampling bias in a survey that uses the internet as a means of data collection.

Central to the success of the use of triangulation as a data collection method is the need for thought to be given to what problems or potential problems the use of triangulated data collection techniques can solve, and what combination of methodologies or methods will best serve to reduce the weakness of any particular approach.

For example, the weakness associated with randomised controlled trials is that they tend to collect quantitative objective data that do not recognise the individuality of the participants or their experience. Increasingly, therefore, medical research into the use of new drugs or interventions has started to include the collection of data about quality of life. While this is not perhaps the truest use of triangulation in research (as quality of life data tend to be collected using quantitative questionnaires), it does acknowledge that the experience of care, for example, taking a new medication or undergoing a new intervention, has to be one that has positive benefits for the patient. These benefits must accrue not only from the medical but also from the human point of view.

What is noteworthy is that for a drug or intervention to be of benefit to people, it must be not only effective but also acceptable to the people affected by it. That is to say, the people who will have to take the medication or be subjected to the intervention must regard its benefits as outweighing any potential or actual side effects (Gomm, 2000a).

There are a number of approaches to triangulation that all serve not only to enrich the quality of the data collected but also to verify it is a true reflection of reality (i.e. it is valid), as the participants see and experience it. These include layering data collection so that the different approaches to data collection become progressively more detailed or probing in what they seek to elicit. So, for example, a brief questionnaire might lead to a focus group, which might lead to a one to one interview. Using such techniques not only allows the richness of the data collected to be increased but also enables the weaknesses of the individual methods to be compensated for. An example might include understanding the quality of life of patients on dialysis. A questionnaire might be used that would elicit some quantitative data. This data might then be explored in the focus group setting where participants could elaborate on some of the issues raised in the questionnaire. Further individuals, perhaps those most or least typical in their contribution in the focus group, might be interviewed one to one to gain even more detail.

Lukkarinen (2005) used questionnaires to ascertain the Health Related Quality of Life (HRQoL) of 280 patients in a study following their treatment for coronary artery disease. Subsequently 19 of the original group underwent qualitative interviews in order to gain a more in-depth understanding of the scores attained during the HRQoL questionnaire phase of the study. This triangulation of the study enabled Lukkarinen to describe the reasons for the differences in the answers to the HRQoL questionnaire given by different groups in the initial phase of the study with a degree of confidence because a number of the respondents themselves had been engaged in the process of explaining the initial findings. This use of triangulation, with questionnaires and interviews, demonstrates how the use of methods of data collection from within the two research paradigms (qualitative and quantitative research) can be used to enhance the validity of a study.

In her study of the use of immunosuppressants in the management of inflammatory bowel disease, Holbrook (2007) collected data on the value of the information given to patients at the start of the new treatment regime from the point of view of the patients and the doctors involved. This provided triangulation about the value of the information given from two different perspectives and therefore provides useful insights into the quality of the information sharing process. In tandem with using triangulation of sources of data – patients and doctors – the data collection included questionnaires with space for the respondents to provide free text clarification of their answers (that is, respondents are allowed to elaborate on their answers using their own words). This free text was used to explore the reasoning behind the answers given and provided a reference point for understanding why respondents had answered in the way they had – that is, it triangulated the data collected.

As well as methodological and methods-based triangulation, there can also be theoretical triangulation within a study. Theoretical triangulation occurs when the underlying philosophy of the research is informed by more than one school of thought. For example, the **structuralist** view of ward life may be more focused on the nurses or the patients as a group in terms of the relationships between them and how they interact. From a structuralist viewpoint the culture of an organisation is understood through studying the policies, management structures and designated roles that influence the relationships of people within it. Whereas, from an **interactionist** viewpoint, the culture of an organisation is understood through studying how people interact in relationships, negotiate their respective roles, and comply with or deviate from what is expected of them.

Theoretical triangulation is therefore about exploring a concept, experience, attitude or interaction from more than one standpoint and, like methodological triangulation, it is about gaining multiple insights into the same issue by taking more than one philosophical starting point. Practically, this is achieved by using more than one data collection method. Ones that allow structuralist exploration might include applying an ethnographic methodology or the collection of data by observation or focus groups, while interactionist examination might require individual interviews.

Fundamental to the success of triangulation is that the blend of approaches used to collect data complement and supplement each other in a reasoned and thought-out way. This requires the researcher to have a good grasp of the pros and cons of each of the methodologies and methods that can be used in nursing research, and to be open to the idea that no single approach to research in nursing practice can be said to hold all of the answers.

> **Concept summary: triangulation**
>
> It may be helpful to use the metaphor of a map to think about triangulation of research methodologies and methods. If you want to tell other people where you are, providing only the longitudinal co-ordinates provides little idea of where you are. But when you provide the latitudinal co-ordinates as well, it is easy for others to find you. In a similar sense, the use of triangulated research methods enhances the ability of researchers not only to find out in more detail what the reality of whatever they are researching is but to communicate these findings with increased accuracy and confidence to others.

So we can view the use of triangulated research as a means of adding a further dimension to research. This additional dimension improves validity by demonstrating that what has been measured is actually a good representation of what we set out to measure. Triangulation also improves reliability by demonstrating that what has been measured and characterised in the research has been shown to hold true when measured in more than one way.

Evaluation research

Evaluation research as a methodology is used to measure the worth or merit of something. It employs any of the methods that have been highlighted in the previous chapters of the book. The key difference lies in the fact that evaluation research occurs within an organisational context, such as a hospital, ward or healthcare team, and it therefore requires the researcher to exercise great diplomatic skills. The nature of evaluative research is such that it requires the involvement of multiple stakeholders whose social, political, professional and personal sensitivities have not only to be recognised but also to be respected.

Evaluation research is a systematic undertaking, and the object of the evaluation can be defined in many different ways. As such, the object of the evaluation may be a programme of care, a care process, the functioning of the ward or care area, the people within the organisation or team, the key activities of the team or organisation, or any combination of the above.

Much of the literature in this area reflects that the evaluation aspect of evaluation research often has as much – if not more – to do with the quality and usefulness of the data it collects as it has to do with the usefulness or merit of the objects, people or processes it is evaluating.

The goal of evaluation research is, therefore, to derive findings that can be used to drive change. The change that ensues has to be driven by the findings of the evaluation and seen to be driven by in-depth empirical investigation of the object of evaluation and not the 'second-hand' application of evidence derived from some study.

Activity 6.2 — *Critical thinking*

Consider some of the questions we have asked about the adoption of research in the area in which you work. What are the issues that derive from research that is undertaken in a different social, political or cultural setting? How do these affect the applicability of research to different settings? How might focused evaluation research be helpful in overcoming some of these issues?

There are some possible answers at the end of the chapter.

You might rightly question why evaluation of a service or process should fall under the umbrella of research rather than audit. Booth (2009) provides four good reasons why evaluation through research rather than evaluative audit is important.

1. Service evaluation tends to be more descriptive and less analytical when undertaken as an audit.
2. Evaluation research helps in the pursuit of an actual answer to the question of quality rather than the generation of further questions that might need further research and do not resolve issues in practice.
3. Evaluation research is more likely to generate statistically tested outcomes that show cause and effect than a local evaluation audit, which will produce statistics that describe only the magnitude of the issue.
4. Evaluation research is more likely to generate findings that can be applied elsewhere (they are generalisable) than a purely locally based evaluation of a service, thus adding to the body of knowledge in an area for the benefit of all.

The use of evaluation research, therefore, has many benefits over and above a pure service evaluation/audit. Service evaluations by their very nature can be threatening to the people who provide the service. They have the potential to discover that the service provided needs improvement or that it is failing in some areas. Undertaking evaluation research, on the other hand, not only provides credibility for the methods used to collect the data, through the application of rigorous research methods, but also means that the ethical principles that apply to the generation of knowledge through research are adhered to (Robson, 2006).

The necessity for evaluation research is well established in the healthcare setting where the worth of what we do as nurses needs to be demonstrated. Not only is this a matter of the clinical, ethical and human imperative of doing the best for our patients, it also arises out of the need to demonstrate that we are making the best use of the resources available. Given the diversity of reasons for undertaking evaluation research, it follows that the methods employed within evaluation research are not restricted to either qualitative or quantitative approaches; rather, the methods that best fit the needs and purposes of the evaluation are applied. As such, evaluation research, with its focus on assessing the usefulness or value of something, can draw on methods from either, or both, research paradigms.

In their evaluation study of the use of ceiling-mounted hoists, Alamgir et al. (2009) demonstrated a good clinical reason for the use of the hoists in reducing the incidence of pressure sores, as well as showing that the hoists had the approval of the patients using them (via qualitative semi-structured interviews). Such an evaluation demonstrates the usefulness of combining the quantitative and qualitative paradigms in order to prove the worth of a change to care provision.

Starting evaluation research

Evaluating the context within which an evaluation takes place is perhaps the most important step in the evaluation research process and is a step that is often undertaken implicitly but not discussed within either the research or the research textbooks.

Context evaluation requires the environment within which the evaluation is to take place to be fully explored and understood before the process of evaluation takes place. There are many factors that impact on the evaluation of the delivery of care. These include issues from the social, political and economic climate within which care is provided as well as the characteristics of the people involved in the delivery and receipt of care.

As such, an evaluation of the context of care will identify the limitations that are placed on the process of the evaluation research. Evaluating the context of the evaluation research also enables the researcher to identify the people who are the stakeholders – people affecting and affected by whatever is being evaluated. Understanding the context of the research, and the nature and variety of the stakeholders will enable the researcher to make informed choices about the approaches they will adopt in the evaluation research study.

Types of evaluation research

Needs assessment

Needs assessment might be used to evaluate whether there is a need for the provision of a new programme of care or a change to a programme currently being provided. The needs assessment may then be used both to substantiate the need for the new or changed programme and also in the design of a programme. Needs assessments are not an evaluation of an existing service or programme of care; they are a means of identifying and quantifying the potential need for a future service.

A needs assessment may be useful in helping to gain approval and funding for a new service. Its purpose is to help identify what needs the new service can be used to meet, as well as identifying those people who might most benefit from the new service.

For example, it is well documented that the uptake of haemodialysis services is highest in areas where a dialysis unit is situated. This tends to suggest that if people live some distance from a dialysis unit, they opt not to have haemodialysis, are not given the option of haemodialysis or choose peritoneal dialysis (usually home based). A needs assessment of the requirement for a new dialysis unit might therefore take into account the positioning of existing units as well as the numbers and geographical locations of people with known established renal failure. It would also consider the demographic characteristics of the population within a location, especially where these characteristics are known to increase the risks for developing renal disease.

Process evaluation

Process evaluations are designed to demonstrate whether a new or changed programme has been implemented in the manner in which it was conceived, as well as examining whether the people accessing the service believe it to be of benefit. The sort of data collected in a process evaluation may include the number of people that use the service and what services they actually received. There is also a qualitative element to this evaluation in that the users of the new service are asked to evaluate its usefulness to them.

For example, in the case of the new dialysis unit described above, there would be evaluations of the numbers of people using the service and what service they actually receive, as well as the impact of the delivery of the new service on the patients' perception of the quality of the care provided to them. Clearly, such an evaluation would take into account both quantitative and qualitative data, which could be collected using a variety of methods.

Formative evaluation

Much in the same way that the progress of student nurses is evaluated part-way through their time on a placement in order to inform them what they need to do to improve, formative evaluations of a service use data gathered during the early phases of the new service to help inform and modify the way in which the service develops. Plainly, these data will include both quantitative and qualitative elements and will reflect the nature of the service being provided.

For example, soon after opening a new dialysis unit, an evaluation of the uptake of the service against that predicted in the initial needs assessment would give some idea of whether the new service is likely to meet its aspirations.

Summative evaluation

Sometimes referred to as an outcome evaluation, summative evaluation is used to measure whether the aims of the service provided have actually been met. This is, again, similar to the summative evaluation given to student nurses at the end of their clinical placement, where they reflect on the objectives that they had been set to see if they have managed to achieve them during the placement.

What is clear is that summative evaluation research looks back at the objectives and aims set at the start of the programme or service and uses these as a benchmark against which delivery is measured. For example, an evaluation of a new dialysis service some months after it opened would give an indication of whether it has progressed from the formative evaluation towards meeting the targets set for the service.

Efficiency evaluation

These evaluations are sometimes called 'cost-effectiveness' or 'cost-benefit valuations'. The purpose of efficiency evaluation research is to examine whether the new service provides good value for money in meeting the objectives that were set for it at the start. For example, a new dialysis unit might be evaluated to see whether it is saving transport costs by treating patients nearer to home, and whether these savings offset the costs of providing the service in the additional location. The important issues with this type of evaluation are not always purely financial but, rather, whether the benefits of the service match up to, or preferably surpass, the money spent. In the case of the haemodialysis patient who has to dialyse three times a week for three to four hours, this benefit may accrue from considerably reduced travelling times and a more personal service in a smaller unit.

Utilisation evaluation

The final type of evaluation research discussed here is utilisation evaluation research. The purpose of this type of evaluation research is to appraise whether the evaluations of the new service or programme have actually been used. It is clear that this type of evaluation research seeks to ascertain whether good practice in the delivery of care persists beyond the end of a programme of initial evaluation.

In nursing we are all aware of the fact that standards and practices change over time and often not always for the right reasons. Many useful evaluations of services are dropped because policy makers or managers have decided that they cannot be afforded or because the levels of motivation within the service delivery team are low.

Utilisation evaluations seek to reinvigorate services by reconnecting the people delivering the service with the quality measures of that service. The purpose is to ensure that the findings of previous evaluation, audit and research are being used to inform the delivery of care.

Utilisation evaluation research is potentially an important aspect of clinical effectiveness and governance. The focus of utilisation evaluation research on measuring the uptake and utilisation of previous findings makes it a clear source of information to informed evidence-based nursing practice in a way that reflects the ESC skill highlighted at the start of the chapter. As such, it is potentially an important research tool for the clinically based nurse.

Action research

Key features

Action research delivers exactly what it says. Action research is research in and on action. The purpose of the inquiry of action research is improvement in the quality of the actions and performance of an organisation, team or individual. The central tenet of the action research approach is that it involves, or preferably is driven by, the people whom it most affects – the key stakeholders – who in the context of this book are often the nurses who work in a specific team or organisation and their patients.

Because of the team approach to undertaking action research, it is often termed a collaborative enquiry. The scope of the team involved in the collaborative enquiry extends beyond the immediate team to all of the individuals who affect, and are affected by, what the team does.

Activity 6.3   *Reflection*

Thinking about the scope of the inquiry associated with action research, take a few moments to think about all of the people who are involved in the delivery and receipt of care where you work at present. Be careful to include all of the people whose roles, however menial they may appear, have an impact not only on the quality of what you do in terms of patients' physical outcomes but also on their experience of care.

There are some possible answers at the end of the chapter.

The purpose and focus of action research is to produce realistic and sustainable improvements in the delivery of care in the setting in which the action research takes place. It allows the providers of the care to reflect on what they do, how they do it and why. It also allows them to explore potential new methods for the delivery of care along with the potential benefits and pitfalls that might accrue from this. The collaborative nature of the process means that the insights and ideas generated are open for sharing and discussion with all of the stakeholders in the process, and the decisions that are therefore made about changes to, and improvements in practice are, potentially, reached through true consensus.

In their action research project aimed at improving end-of-life care of elderly residents of care facilities, Rowley and Taylor (2011) adopted a six-phase approach. The phases applied during the research were: foundation building (recruiting participants and explaining the process); reflections on practice stories (sharing experiences); learning from the relatives (the use of anonymised interviews to aid deeper reflection); identifying thematic concerns (core areas of interest for the participants and their work areas); action plan creation and implementation (how the team were going to address the care concerns raised); and critical reflection on action (consideration of the impact of the plan). This approach to the project enabled the researchers to generate what they considered to be a sustainable and practical model for improving pain management in terminally ill residents of elderly care facilities.

The British tradition of action research echoes the view of action research as research that is focused on the direct improvement of practice. This tradition is firmly grounded in reflection. Classic action research is described by Carr and Kemmis (1986, p162) as *simply a form of self-reflective enquiry undertaken by participants in social situations in order to improve the rationality and justice of their own practices, their understanding of these practices, and the situations in which the practices are carried out.*

As such, this form of action research is attractive to nurses, who are practised in reflection from working in the academic and clinical setting.

The action research cycle

The need for an action research project often arises out of the realisation that there is an issue in practice that needs addressing but for which there appears to be no readily identifiable solution.

Lewin (1946), who coined the phrase 'action research', created the cycle of action research (see Figure 6.1), which is still guiding many action researchers to date. Many researchers refer to the cycle as the methodology which guides action research. The adoption of the cycle as a map for action research is, however, probably a misinterpretation of the purpose of the cycle, which is more of a guide than a methodological blueprint.

The recurring cycles of action research produce spiral cycles of action research, with the researcher re-entering the cycle to address new issues that arise during the implementation of the action phases.

This action research cycle is often stated as being 'reflect, plan, act, observe, reflect . . .' and, as such, mirrors in many ways the nursing process of 'assess, plan, implement and evaluate'. The

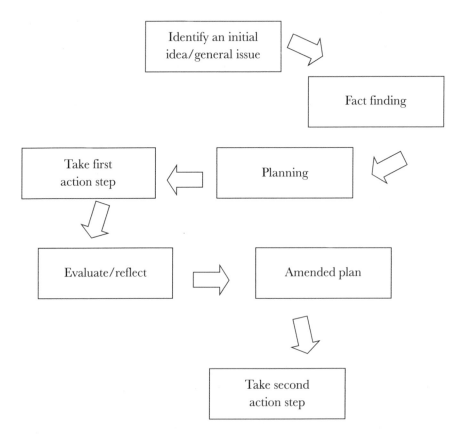

Figure 6.1: The action research cycle

Source: adapted from Lewin (1946).

starting point for a piece of action research can be any point within this cycle. For instance, the realisation of the need for change might arise out of reflection on a clinical incident or issue, or the need to implement a new externally imposed process, policy or procedure that requires some changes in the way in which the team or organisation works.

In their five-year, three-cycle study that set out to empower patients with dementia, Nomura et al. (2009) used a variety of strategies to increase the integration of people with dementia at an individual, group and community level. The strategies for integration were developed as a result of observational data collection, written comments collected from caregivers, and records of phone interviews and counselling with caregivers. This action research demonstrates the spiralling cyclical process through which action research develops a programme or process while using a variety of data collection strategies among a number of stakeholders in order to validate the research.

What makes action research such a challenge to undertake is that there is often more than one spiral of action underway at any time. This means that researchers engaged in action research may be reflecting on the impact of one action while simultaneously implementing another.

The process of action research relies more on democracy, reflexivity, change and collaboration than slavishly following a prescribed methodology. Because of its agenda of affecting meaningful and lasting change, there is a requirement that action research meets the needs of all of the people involved and that all the people it affects are involved (democracy and collaboration).

Given the involvement of the researchers in the process and because the very presence of the researchers has an impact on the process, there is a requirement that as well as being reflective, the researchers are also reflexive. Reflexivity requires researchers to be open to and understand the impact of their presence, their actions and the choices that they make on the process of the research.

Data collection methods

The methods used for the collection of data within action research are restricted only by the imagination and skills of the people undertaking the research. As a methodology, action research is not bounded by the philosophies and conventions associated with the quantitative or qualitative paradigms. The purpose of action research is the instigation of change and the development of the organisation, team or process. This cannot be subject to the artificial and somewhat divisive conventions of the two research paradigms.

Data collection within action research requires not only that the issue under investigation is understood but also that data are collected so that the nature of the plan, actions derived from the plan and the subsequent evaluation and reflection on the action are coherently and compre-hensively understood.

This means that data collection within action research is driven more by the nature of the individual questions that arise than by the paradigm within which it sits. Typical data collection strategies, therefore, include surveys, questionnaires, interviews, focus groups, examination of existing records and observation. As within the traditional paradigms and their associated methodologies and methods, thought needs to be given to which approaches to data collection are likely to produce the data that are needed to meet the aims of the research. An action research project is not restricted to the use of one method of data collection; rather, the different phases of the action research process may require different methodological approaches and methods of data collection, depending on the particular problem being addressed.

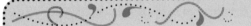

Chapter summary

This chapter has established that adherence to the strict delineations of qualitative or quantitative research methodologies may not always be the best approach to answering complex questions arising out of the delivery of nursing care. We have established that understanding and delivering good quality care requires us to understand not only the physical and psychological aspects of care but also the emotional aspects and how the care is experienced.

Triangulation has been highlighted as one way in which the philosophy, methodology and methods of research can be reconciled so that more than one dimension of a problem can be explored. We see that by viewing a research issue from more than one standpoint, the understanding that can be gained is both deeper and better defined.

We have seen that evaluation research allows for the appraisal of a team, an organisation or a programme of care. We have seen that evaluation is bounded to a time and a place and is designed to answer questions about the area being researched. Evaluation research is therefore portrayed as a helpful means of collecting data that are perhaps more meaningful than those collected by some forms of clinical audit, in effecting meaningful change.

We also discussed the nature of action research – unusual among the research methodologies in that the subjects of the research are also intimately involved in the research. We have seen that action research rarely follows a predetermined methodology; rather, it is responsive to its own findings and adapts as it goes along.

Activities: Brief outline answers

Activity 6.2: Critical thinking (page 119)

Research undertaken in different settings is affected by the demographic make-up of the population from which the sample for the research is drawn. The way in which the sample is selected also has potential to affect the applicability of the research findings to the clinical setting. Evaluation research undertaken in the area in which the findings are to be applied overcomes these issues as it draws its sample from the same population the research will take place in.

Activity 6.3: Reflection (page 123)

Potential stakeholders in action research in the care setting are:

- nurses;
- students;

- doctors;
- allied health professionals;
- support staff;
- patients;
- patients' relatives;
- voluntary staff;
- the community at large.

Further reading

Clarke, E (2001) Evaluation research in nursing and healthcare. *Nurse Researcher*. 8 (3): 4–14.

An overview of healthcare evaluation research methods as they apply to nursing.

McNiff, J and Whitehead, AJ (2009) *Doing and writing action research*. London: Sage.

A comprehensive and user-friendly guide to action research.

Meyer, J (2006) Action research, in Gerish, K and Lacey, A (eds) *The research process in nursing* (5th edn). Oxford: Blackwell.

Robson, C (2006) Evaluation research, in Gerish, K and Lacey, A (eds) *The research process in nursing* (5th edn). Oxford: Blackwell.

Streubert Speziale, HJ and Carpenter, DR (2007) *Qualitative research in nursing: advancing the humanistic imperative* (4th edn). London: Lippincott Williams & Wilkins.

Chapter 15, Triangulation as a qualitative research strategy, gives a brief but informative overview of this subject area.

Useful websites

www.did.stu.mmu.ac.uk/carnnew/ The Collaborative Action Research Network (see the resources tab for other useful links).

www.hta.ac.uk/ The National Institute for Health Research's Health Technology Assessment Programme website. This website provides an insight into the evaluation of effectiveness, costs and impact of healthcare interventions.

www.jeanmcniff.com Look under the 'booklet' tab for a brief and simple to read overview introduction to action research from a leading exponent of action research.

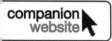 For further activities and other useful material, visit the companion website at **www.sagepub.co.uk/ellis_research2e**

apter 7
using research

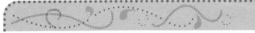

NMC Standards for Pre-registration Nursing Education

This chapter will address the following competencies:

Domain 1: Professional values

7. All nurses must be responsible and accountable for keeping their knowledge and skills up to date through continuing professional development. They must aim to improve their performance and enhance the safety and quality of care through evaluation, supervision and appraisal.
8. All nurses must practise independently, recognising the limits of their competence and knowledge. They must reflect on these limits and seek advice from, or refer to, other professionals where necessary.
9. All nurses must appreciate the value of evidence in practice, be able to understand and appraise research, apply relevant theory and research findings to their work, and identify areas for further investigation.

Domain 4: Leadership, management and team working

1. All nurses must act as change agents and provide leadership through quality improvement and service development to enhance people's wellbeing and experiences of healthcare.
2. All nurses must systematically evaluate care and ensure that they and others use the findings to help improve people's experience and care outcomes and to shape future services.

NMC Essential Skills Clusters

This chapter will address the following ESC:

Organisational aspects of care

16. People can trust the newly registered graduate nurse to safely lead, co-ordinate and manage care.

Introduction

So far this book has introduced you to the main paradigms, methodologies, methods, etc. associated with undertaking research in a nursing context. For some readers this will have been a journey of necessity, for example because you are taking a research module at university, while for others this will have been purely through an interest in the subject area of research; in reality the reason for writing this book has been to address, at least in part, both of these. Of course, the main motive for being interested in research and research practice for all exponents of health and social care, and the reason this book was written, is the recognition of the positive impact that research can have on the health and well-being of people.

In this deliberately brief chapter, we will consider how we might use the content of the rest of the book to address a number of your needs as a student both in the immediate term (to pass assignments and plan projects) and in the long term to deliver informed and judicious care.

Why research is important

Elsewhere in this series Ellis (2013) presents an extended argument as to why the use of evidence in nursing practice is important. There are some key reasons as to why the use of evidence-based practice is important that are worth reiterating here.

The key starting point is to understand knowledge changes over time. What we think we 'know' today might be shown to be wrong tomorrow as human understanding and technologies for understanding the world develop. This means we cannot rest on our laurels, we have to engage with nursing as a lifelong learning exercise, developing what we do and how we do it to reflect the needs of society, patients and clients as well as the current state of knowledge. In some cases this will be appreciating and adopting a new approach to treating some disease or disability (as we saw in the quantitative chapters); while in others (as we have seen in the chapters on qualitative research) it will be about understanding how people experience their treatment and the care we provide. Either way, as individuals we can make the choice either just to adopt the changes because we have been told to do so, or we can try to understand, or indeed introduce, the changes ourselves.

However we choose to view it, using research is an integral part of the role of the nurse. There is a moral imperative for us to provide the best care we can for our clients and patients, and this means at a minimum being able to understand what is good and what is bad in the research we read, and therefore how much faith we place in it prior to adopting it in practice.

A good deal of what health and social care practitioners do is not research based, but then most health and social care commentators now agree that evidence-based practice, widely agreed to be the proper way to provide care, is not, cannot and will never be entirely research driven. There are a number of good reasons why this is the case, as shown below.

Why research and evidence-based care are not synonymous

- Not everything can be researched.
- Not everything has been researched.
- Not all situations are identical and therefore existing research may not apply.
- Researched outcomes only apply to broadly similar situations.
- People have the right to make non-research-based choices.

What the above list demonstrates is that there are many influences on the decisions we make as nurses and there are many reasons why research may not always inform practice. Ellis (2013) lists a number of influences on the decisions we make in practice:

- research evidence;
- practice knowledge;
- experience;
- policy;
- resources;
- patient preference;
- views of other professionals;
- ethics;
- law.

Evidently, these influences are of differing levels of importance depending on the scenario to which they are being applied but, and this is an important but, of the influences on practice research evidence is, when of good quality, the most reliable and readily justifiable. Each of the other influences on practice, while important as a consideration for how and why we might act, is open to opinion and individual interpretation.

The NMC competencies highlighted at the start of this chapter exhort us to take responsibility for our actions as nurses, to act independently while appreciating the value of evidence. The competencies also go further in requiring practising nurses to act as agents for change (or perhaps more correctly improvement) in order that the experiences and outcomes of care of our patients are continually improving.

These are lofty ideals and as we move towards an era of all graduate nurses and the associated increased professionalisation of nursing the importance of these competencies becomes more evident.

The rest of this chapter will explore a little of how research can be used to inform both practice situations and academic work. The reader is advised to look elsewhere for more in-depth discussion and analysis of the other available, and valid, approaches to decision making (see Further reading).

Using research to inform practice

Getting research into practice involves a number of key steps. One of the first things we need to be clear about is the fact that not all research is good, not all research comes to the right conclusions and not all research will necessarily apply to the situation before us.

Hek and Moule (2011) suggest a very useful route plan for the adoption of evidence in practice using five distinct but connected stages. Of note, each of the stages requires the nurse to be critical not only of the evidence presented but also within each of the stages of the process.

1. Identify a problem from practice and turn it into a specific question.
2. Find the best available evidence that relates to the question, usually by systematically searching the literature.
3. Appraise the evidence.
4. Identify the best evidence alongside the patient's needs and preferences.
5. Evaluate the effect of applying the evidence.

The rest of this chapter will essentially use this five-stage model to inform our thinking about how we might use research either for an academic undertaking or to improve practice.

Stages 1 to 3 provide a useful blueprint for many academic undertakings such as critiquing literature within an evidence-based practice or research module or in the process of designing a piece of research. Good academic practice in general requires the explicit and thoughtful use of research to inform any essay or assignment, and this will include being critical about its quality. The discussion that follows about these first three stages will therefore be helpful in the planning and execution of such undertakings, but the reader is advised to look elsewhere to extend and supplement their understanding as well (see Further reading).

Of course, not all academic work is specifically about designing or critiquing research studies; there are many other occasions when the use of research in an essay is needed. Any academic paper that has a clinical element to it should be informed by the use of research and more specifically journal-based literature. There are two good reasons for this: the first is that clinical textbooks become out of date quickly as new advances in care delivery are discovered and therefore your development as a practitioner *must* be supplemented by an understanding of current best practice. The second reason is that it demonstrates your ability to identify and engage with lifelong learning and as such will impress the marker!

As with all academic undertakings, it is not enough merely to cite or quote research; the best students will also include some description of the context of the research and perhaps a critique of the methodology/methods as well. Such critique demonstrates the ability to understand the context of research and independent thinking.

If you are considering how you might use research to inform and better practise, all five stages of the model are of benefit, and again you are advised to use further literature to inform your thinking in this area (see Further reading).

Generating a specific question

Generating a specific question relating to a clinical situation is not always as easy as it might seem. In Chapter 1 we explored the use of the acronyms SPICE and PICO to enable us to generate questions that are clear, focused and relevant.

Activity 7.1   *Reflection*

Review the section in Chapter 1 entitled 'Developing research questions' (pages 8–11). Consider your answers to Activities 1.2 and 1.3 and therefore what a good research question should look like.

As the answer is based on your own reflection, there is no outline answer at the end of the chapter.

Once we have identified our practice problem and turned it into a useful question there is increased clarity about what exactly we are trying to achieve. For example, are we looking for a hard-and-fast scientific answer to a medical, technical or measurable issue or are we trying to understand the opinion, attitudes or beliefs that inform a behaviour or response to treatment? This in turn helps us to identify which of the two paradigms (or potentially mixed methodology) of research we should be exploring. Table 2.3 in Chapter 2 and Table 4.1 in Chapter 4 provide some insight into the types of question different research approaches might be able to answer.

Finding the best available evidence

When we have a useful question we are ready to take the next step in the process, which is to search the literature (see the chapter on 'Sources of knowledge for evidence-based care' in Ellis (2013)).

There are some key important issues about finding evidence that are worth considering here. Importantly, just because something is in print, on the web or has been told to you does not mean it is necessarily right. The first clue we might gather as to the usefulness of a source of information is the quality of the resource itself. Looking for information to inform practice in a general newspaper or an unmoderated website is most certainly not a good idea. Quality sources of information for nursing include those websites and journals that are peer reviewed (that is, where the content has been reviewed by other specialists in the field to confirm its quality). For the most part such sources will be aimed at a professional audience, which may include nurses and other health and social care professionals; this is, of course, subject dependent.

Good-quality journals can be searched using bibliographic databases such as CINAHL (Cumulative Index of Nursing and Allied Health Literature) and the British Nursing Index. Using the terminology identified in the generation of the question is step one, followed by the use of other key words that are focused on the topic in hand. Learning to search bibliographic databases effectively is a good skill to have for either academic or clinical purposes; all universities and many hospital libraries will provide workshops on how to do this effectively.

Appraising the evidence

This is the real crux of the whole process. Understanding research, hence the name of this book, requires engagement with reading and comprehension of the research process. Whatever you are reading research for, the stages involved in its appraisal and the tools you will need remain the same. As well as using a critiquing framework (see, for example, Ellis (2013), a snippet of which is provided later) for effective evaluation of research, you will also need to hand at least one good research textbook, which you can use as a reference as to what good research looks like.

One of the key errors students make when critiquing research is to think the use of a word in research is synonymous with the use of the word in everyday life. This means they often fail to appreciate what a framework is asking them to do, *critique*. For example, the use of the term 'bias' in research is, as we have seen elsewhere in the book, very specific, therefore applying the term in its everyday sense is not what is required. So tip two for effective critiquing is to use a glossary to ensure you understand and apply critiquing terms effectively. Getting the critique right will also impact on the potential clinical application of a research paper where, for example, selection biases may mean that a study is not pertinent to the patients you are caring for – that is, the findings are not generalisable or transferable.

Activity 7.2   *Evidence-based practice and research*

Consider the use of the term 'reliability' in everyday life. What does it mean and in what contexts might you use it? Now research the meaning of reliability in relation to research – what does it mean and in what contexts does it apply?

As this activity is based on your own reflection, there is no outline answer at the end of the chapter.

This idea of the use of research terminology in critiquing leads us to a third tip in relation to successful critiquing, especially in the academic sense. In an essay or other written assignment you only have one opportunity to get your point across and to let the marker know that you know what it is you are talking about. So, to ensure you make this communication effectively it is useful to *define* your terms, *reference* the definition and then *apply* the definition to the critique.

> **Concept summary: defining, referencing and applying a research definition**
>
> For example, you might say that in qualitative research the term 'trustworthiness' is used to refer to the quality of the procedures used in the process of undertaking the research; this is your *definition*. You might then *reference* this definition to a good-quality, pertinent research textbook. You would then *apply* the definition to the critique by saying whatever it is you wanted to say about the quality of the research procedures used in the research in question.

In the academic sense it is then important to critique the elements of the paper you are asked to critique; no more and no less. Often academic critiques focus on elements of the question asked, the paradigm, methodology and methods chosen. A good critique will examine each of these in turn with reference to a research textbook to define what they are and the pros and cons of each. Again in the academic setting, it may be important to suggest alternative ways of answering the same question (although for practical applications of research critiquing this may not be so important). So, for example, the critiquing framework by Ellis (2013) suggests asking the following question.

- Given the methodology identified (if any), do the research data collection methods fit?
  - Even if yes, are there alternative methods that might be appropriate as well?

Providing a full answer to this demonstrates to the marker that you understand not only how to critique what is in front of you, but also the range of techniques available to collect data in similar situations, that is to say, you understand the broader research process.

Using the best evidence and considering patient preference

In the practice setting the use of evidence is about the way in which we, as nurses, respond to the reality of the patient's situation. That means our critique of evidence provides only one step of the process in clinical decision making.

Perhaps the most widely quoted definition comes from Sackett et al. (1996, p71), who defined evidence-based medicine as:

> *the conscientious, explicit and judicious use of current best evidence in making decisions about the care of the individual patient. It means integrating individual clinical expertise with the best available external clinical evidence from systematic research.*

What Sackett et al. are saying here is that we need to ensure the decisions we make are guided by thoughtful processes that are guided by both explicit forms of evidence (such as research) and the requirements of the individual patient. It does not matter that this definition is about medicine, since the same ideas translate to the adoption of evidence in nursing practice.

Of course, we have to make other judgements about research and other forms of evidence in the context of our practice before we consider if, when and how we might apply it. Gomm (2000a, p171) asks the pertinent question, *Would it work here?*. In asking this question Gomm is reminding us that while research is a useful indicator of what good healthcare might look like, we should consider some practicalities. Some questions you might ask when considering the application of research are suggested below.

Questions to ask before adopting research-driven change

- Can we afford the change?
- What are the potential benefits:
  - to patients
  - to staff
  - to the organisation?
- What are the potential disadvantages:
  - to patients
  - to staff
  - to the organisation?
- Are the people in the research broadly similar to the people we will be applying it to?
- What might our patients (current and future) think about this?
- What are the alternatives?
- Do we have the skills necessary, or can we acquire them?
- How will we instigate the change?
- Who will lead the change?

While, in the broadest sense, these are reasonable questions to ask, we might also consider what alternatives might be in place for patients who do not want the change we are considering adopting (e.g. an alteration to a wound-dressing regime or changing the mode of delivery of a medication).

The key message here is that while research is perhaps the most useful tool we have to inform practice, it is not an end in itself. Research in nursing is applied in a context of human interaction and as such needs to consider ability, preference and affordability. Any adoption of research evidence into practice that does not account for these will be more likely to fail than one that does, not least of all because people, nurses included, are very often scared by change (for a broader discussion of this, see *Evidence-based Nursing Practice* (Ellis, 2013), also in this series).

Activity 7.3   *Reflection*

Consider a time when you had to make a change in your life. Perhaps it was moving away from home to go to university or starting on a new practice placement for the first time. Even though these are meant to be positive events, what emotions did you experience? Consider also how you felt making the transition from school to university essay writing. You may have developed a style of writing for school that was effective and brought you success and now you are being asked to relearn something you thought you had already

continued . . .

mastered; what impact did this have on how you felt about yourself and your academic ability?

As the answer is based on your own reflection, there is no outline answer at the end of the chapter.

What you might note on undertaking this reflection is that all change is associated with an emotional response. Changes that impact on how you feel about yourself and your ability can feel very alarming. The essential message here is that the adoption of evidence for practice is not purely an academic process; the need to bring people (patients and staff alike) along on the journey is as important, if not more, than understanding the evidence itself.

Patients are people and in modern society people possess the right to make choices, even if these are *bad* ones, so part of the armoury of the evidence-based nurse is the ability to inform patients of their options and to then work *with* them to make choices that suit their individual circumstances and preferences.

Evaluating the application of evidence

We said early on in the chapter that providing good-quality evidence-driven care is a moral imperative for nurses. Meeting the demands of this moral imperative requires that in the practice setting we evaluate what we have done and its effectiveness; at no time is this more important than after we have made a change to practice.

The purpose of evaluating a change is to answer the question, *Has it worked here?* In some respects evaluating the outcomes of the adoption of evidence in this way injects an air of reality into the process because it answers many of the questions we posed on page 135. Evaluation post-implementation is in many senses more realistic than asking questions before the implementation because we are measuring what *actually* happened, rather than what *might* happen.

Evaluating the implementation of research is also important because, as we have seen, research scenarios are often manipulated to suit the needs of the research itself and therefore they may not represent real life.

The process of evaluating a change is much like the process of undertaking research using the methodology of a quasi- (or natural) experiment (discussed in Chapter 4). Considering the requirements of a natural experiment it is clear that we need to collect data both before and after a change has been implemented in order that we might compare and contrast two approaches to care. So, for example, if we were to alter a care regime we might want to measure the impact of the change on clinical patient outcomes as well as, perhaps, the patient experience.

Case study

In their study to ascertain the impact of changing transfusion practices in the trauma setting, Nakstad et al. (2011) measured the impact of a move towards a more widespread use of haemostatic agents (which promote blood clotting) rather than blood products (which aim only to restore haemoglobin levels). The change to the use of haemostatic agents was a conscious clinical decision and was not undertaken as a result of a study protocol; in that respect this study represents a natural experiment. The key outcome of interest here was patient survival!

Where standards of care already exist, the implementation of a new way of working might be evaluated using an audit, although as we saw in the section on evaluation research (Chapter 6, pages 118–22) audit is often constrained in what it can tell us about how and what to improve.

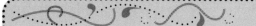

Chapter summary

This chapter is little more than a sample of the debate about evidence-based nursing practice. We have seen in this chapter that the adoption of research evidence is complicated by issues such as: identifying a clinical problem; identifying research to address the problem; assessing the quality of the research; considering the quality and applicability of the research as well as the potential for other forms of evidence; and the need to pay due consideration to the needs and preferences of the individuals the evidence will affect.

Evidently this chapter has established that research is only a means to an end and that end is improved patient care. In this chapter we have further established that the route to improved care lies not in the blind, uninformed acceptance of the findings of research, but in conscientious and informed appraisal of evidence applied thoughtfully and appreciatively.

Further reading

Ellis, P (2013) *Evidence-based Nursing Practice*, 2nd edn. London: Sage/Learning Matters.

See especially the final chapter on getting evidence into practice.

Gomm, R and Davies, C (eds) (2000) *Using Evidence in Health and Social Care*. London: Sage.

A slightly old but very practical book.

National Institute for Health and Clinical Excellence (NICE) (2007) *How to Change Practice: Understand, identify and overcome barriers to change*. London: NICE.

Standing, M (2011) *Clinical Judgement and Decision Making for Nursing Students*. Exeter: Learning Matters.

Guides you through ten aspects of nurses' clinical decision making (e.g. systematic, standardised), which are informed by different types of evidence including research.

Useful websites

www.evidence.nhs.uk Clinical and non-clinical evidence and best practice website from the NHS.

www.nice.org.uk The website of the National Institute for Health and Clinical Excellence.

www.sign.ac.uk The Scottish Intercollegiate Guidelines Network (SIGN) develops evidence-based clinical practice guidelines for the NHS in Scotland.

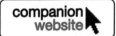

For further activities and other useful material, visit the companion website at **www.sagepub.co.uk/ellis_research2e**

Glossary

anthropology: the study of humans and human behaviours.

association: a potential causal connection between two variables.

autonomy: the ability to make choices for oneself.

average: the common name of the arithmetic mean, which is the sum of all the observations in a data set divided by the number of observations.

behavioural bias: bias that occurs when people within a study behave in a given manner because of some underlying reason that usually affects all similar individuals.

beneficence: the ethical principle of doing good.

bias: in the context of research, anything in the design or undertaking of a study that causes an untruth to occur in the study potentially affecting the outcome of the study. See also measurement bias; recall bias; response bias; selection bias.

blinding: the process of hiding from either the participant (single blind) or both the participant and the researchers (double blind) which arm of a study (usually a randomised controlled trial) a participant is allocated to. Also known as masking.

bracketing: also referred to as epoching the process of putting all of your preconceptions about a topic to one side to allow the exploration of a topic as if you were naive about it. This only applies to some forms of phenomenology.

closed question: a question that requires a limited range of responses such as 'yes' or 'no'.

confounding: occurs when alternative explanations for an outcome in a study are not accounted for. Confounding variables are always independently associated with both the exposure and the outcome being measured. For example, an increased risk of cancer of the pancreas is associated with both smoking and coffee drinking, and smokers tend to drink more coffee than non-smokers.

consequentialist ethics: the school of ethical thought that states that the consequences of an action (achieving the greater good) are more important than the action itself.

control arm: the arm of a randomised controlled trial to which the intervention under research is not applied. People in this arm of an RCT are otherwise treated in the same way as people in the intervention arm. This allows the researchers to be sure that the intervention being studied causes the outcome they are measuring.

convenience sample: a sample taken from a set of individuals who are easily accessed.

correlation: an apparent association (cause and effect) between two variables. A positive correlation occurs in situations when a rise in the independent variable causes an increase in the dependent, while a negative correlation occurs when a rise in the value of the independent variable causes a decrease in the dependent.

credible/credibility: believable. A term used in qualitative research to suggest that the research undertaken actually answers what it set out to answer because of the quality of the way in which the research has been done.

data saturation: the point during data collection for a qualitative study at which no more new ideas or observations are emerging from the people being studied.

deductive: refers to research that sets out to prove an existing idea or hypothesis. The research sets out to explore the truthfulness of the original idea.

dependent variable: the outcome variable of the study that occurs as a result of the independent variable having occurred (also called the outcome).

descriptive phenomenology: the study of the essence of being that seeks to apply no interpretation; that is, phenomenology that literally just describes the phenomenon of interest.

descriptive statistics: statistics used to describe the frequencies and patterns of numbers within a data set.

emic: taking the insider view – seeing the world from someone else's point of view.

empirical: the notion of discovering new things using the senses or, in the case of research, different methods.

epidemiology: the study of diseases and their treatments from a population perspective.

epistemology: the philosophy of knowledge.

epoching: see 'bracketing'.

equivalence studies: comparative studies that compare a new treatment to the current best treatment rather than a placebo.

essence: the nature of something.

etic: the outsider's view of something.

experimental: a way of testing a hypothesis through comparison.

exposure: see 'independent variable'.

gatekeeper: in the research sense, someone from within a group who helps a researcher gain access to the group in order to undertake their study.

generalise/generalisability: refers to the ability of the findings of a study to be extrapolated to the wider population.

Hawthorne effect: occurs when people respond in the manner in which they believe they should when confronted by a researcher asking questions. The Hawthorne effect can bias a study.

hermeneutics: the interpretation and understanding of language.

homogeneous: the same.

hypothesis: an idea that quantitative research sets out to prove.

incidence: the number of new instances of an event (e.g. an illness) in a given period of time. It sounds like the word 'incident' and, indeed, shares the meaning of a new occurrence.

independent variable: the causal variable in a study, which may be manipulated during a study (also called the exposure).

inductive: refers to the process of developing a theory or hypothesis by first collecting and examining the evidence and seeing where this leads.

inferential statistics: statistics that are used to draw conclusions about the level of association between two or more variables within a study.

interactionist: a philosophical approach that is concerned with how individuals view the world and how they operate in it.

interpretative phenomenology: phenomenology that attempts to apply an interpretation or understanding to the data collected from the research participants.

interpretative phenomenological analysis: interpretative phenomenology that takes account of the fact that the interpretation applied is actually an interpretation of the participant's interpretation of their own experience.

interventional: generally applied in quantitative research when an intentional intervention is applied to a research subject in order to measure the effect of the intervention.

justice: to do with acting fairly so that people are treated generally in the same way.

masking see blinding

mean: also called the average; the sum of all the observations in a data set divided by the number of observations.

measurement bias: bias that occurs when something is measured incorrectly in a consistent manner.

median: the middle value of an ordered set of observations.

methodologies: the broad approaches to research that provide the general framework of the enquiry.

methods: in the sense they are used in this book, the specific tools used to collect data during the research process, e.g. a questionnaire.

mode: the most frequently occurring number in a data set.

mortality rate: the death rate in a given population.

non-consequentialist: a view of ethics whereby the action is more important than the outcome. Doing the right thing is therefore seen as more important than what actually happens as a consequence.

non-maleficence: the ethical principle of avoiding doing harm, perhaps better thought of as 'first do no harm'.

null hypothesis: a term whereby a hypothesis is posed as the opposite of what the researchers actually expect to find. Null hypotheses are posed for statistical reasons.

observational studies: studies that involve observation, which in quantitative research is usually quite structured and in qualitative research much less so. Observational studies do not involve an intervention on the part of the researcher.

open question: a question that does not appear to suggest an answer, allowing the respondent to give whatever answer they think of.

outcome: see 'dependent variable'.

paradigm: in the sense that this term is applied in the book, the philosophical position that is taken within the research.

participant observation: observing the functioning of a group from within the group.

phenomenology: a research methodology within qualitative research concerned with understanding an experience from the point of view of someone experiencing the phenomenon of interest.

placebo: an inactive form of a treatment used as a comparison in experiments involving new treatments or interventions.

placebo effect: a potentially noticeable improvement in someone's condition that is not due to any active intervention. The improvement is, in fact, the result of what is probably a psychological response to being paid attention.

prevalence/prevalent: the amount of a disease in a defined population at a given point in time. So if a disease lasts for life, its prevalence will continue to rise, even if the incident rate is low, whereas for a short-lived illness such as a cold or measles the incidence rate and prevalence will be broadly similar. Often people use the two terms interchangeably, but they are not the same thing.

probability sampling: sampling that gives everyone in the study population the same chance of being selected for a study as long as they meet the inclusion criteria. When large enough, such sampling produces results that are generalisable to the population from which the sample is drawn.

prospective: going forward in time.

purposive: refers to a method of sampling within qualitative research whereby people are chosen for inclusion because they meet the purpose of the study. This means they have experience of the phenomenon being studied.

qualitative paradigm: a position associated with the social and psychological sciences. People using this paradigm are interested in discovering truths about how people experience the world and why.

quantitative paradigm: a position that views the world in a more conventionally scientific sense. People using this paradigm are interested in proving associations, correlations and cause and effect.

randomised controlled trial (RCT): a specific form of experiment that is used in the clinical setting in order to compare the usefulness of two or more interventions.

range: the difference between the largest observation of a data set and the smallest observation.

recall bias: bias that occurs when individuals in a study have to rely on their memory in order to answer certain questions. Such biases are created when people who are ill, or have another reason to remember an exposure, are better at recalling events than people who are not ill.

reflexive/reflexivity: the conscious engagement on the part of the researcher in being open to and expressing their own biases and opinions that may affect the carrying out and interpretation of the research.

relevance: in the qualitative sense this refers to the extent to which the findings of a study might be applied outside the context of the original research.

reliability/reliable: refers to whether a method of data collection, or measurement, will repeatedly give the same results if used by the same person more than once or by two or more people when measuring the same phenomenon.

representative: the amount of similarity between a study sample and the population from which it is drawn.

research process: a structured approach to asking a research question that is then addressed in a methodical, structured, scientific manner.

response bias: bias that occurs when individuals respond to a question within a study in a particular way because they think that the answer they are giving is what the researcher wants to hear.

retrospective: looking back in time.

rigour/rigorous: a term used in qualitative research that suggests that the research process has been undertaken in a well thought through, well-explained and transparent manner.

sampling bias: bias that occurs when the selection of a sample for a study may exclude certain groups of people in a systematic manner; for example, an online survey will exclude all those people who do not have internet access.

selection bias: bias as a result of an action occurring on one side of a study and not the other. So if researchers were allowed to decide which participants had which intervention in a study, it is possible that they might select patients they thought would do better in the study or try harder to follow a regime – this would be called selection bias.

semi-structured interview: an interview that is partially guided using something like a topic guide or predetermined list of questions.

sensitivity: a measure of the ability of a test to detect a positive result when a result is in truth positive.

sham treatment/intervention: a fake (placebo) treatment used as a comparison for a new treatment in an experiment such as a randomised controlled trial.

structuralist: a philosophical approach concerned with how individuals behave within a group, allowing an understanding of how group cultures are formed and operate.

subjective: a word used to demonstrate that people see the world in different ways, from their own personal perspective.

symbolic interactionism: the study of micro-scale social interactions.

tacit knowledge: knowledge that is so deeply embedded that people often forget they have it. It is known to people within a group and does not need explanation within the context of that group, but may be unknown to outsiders.

temporal effect: an effect that makes sense over a period of time such as a reduction in pain over the few minutes following a kick to the shin.

theoretical sampling: a method of sampling that occurs as researchers build new theories and ideas from the data they have collected and test these theories by interviewing more subjects to see if the new theories still hold true. Usually only a feature of grounded theory research. Also called 'handy sampling'.

theory: an understanding about an issue that has been derived by collecting evidence.

topic guides: short lists of questions to be used as a way of keeping the interviewer focused on the purpose of the interview while also allowing some flexibility.

uncertainty principle: the starting point for all research – because we are uncertain about the answer to a specific question, we undertake research in order to try to remove the uncertainty.

unstructured interview: an interview that is conducted with few if any guiding questions. These interviews are usually very exploratory in nature.

utilitarian ethics: a school of ethical thought that states that the consequences of an action (achieving the greater good) are more important than the action itself.

validity / valid: refers to the ability of a method (or data collection technique) to measure what it is supposed to be measuring. For example, we know that a thermometer (if placed correctly for long enough) will measure temperature, but it is not easy to be certain that a questionnaire designed to measure quality of life actually does so because of the difficulty of defining what quality of life actually is.

variable: literally something that varies, such as eye colour or age. In the sense of research it refers to the thing being explored within the study.

verbatim: word for word, literally 'as something was said'.

References

Alamgir, H, Li, OW, Gorman, E, Fast, C, Schicheng, Y and Kidd, C (2009) Professional practice evaluation of ceiling lifts in health care settings: patient outcome and perceptions. *American Association of Occupational Health Nurses Journal*, 57 (9): 374–80.

Al-Farsi, YM, Al-Shabati, MM, Waly, MI, Al-Farsi, OA, Al-Shafaee, MA, Al-Khaduri, MM et al. (2012) Effects of sub-optimal breast-feeding on occurrence of autism: a case-control study. Nutrition, 28 (7/8): e27–e32.

Altman, DG (1991) *Practical statistics for medical research*. London: Chapman and Hall.

Beauchamp, T and Childress, J (2008) *Principles of biomedical ethics* (6th edn). Oxford: Oxford University Press.

Bland, JM and Altman, DG (1994) Regression towards the mean. *British Medical Journal*, 308: 1499.

Booth, A (2009) Using evidence in practice: research or evaluation? Does it matter? *Health Information and Libraries Journal*, 26: 255–8.

Bradbury-Jones, C, Sambrook, S and Irvine, F (2009) The phenomenological focus group: an oxymoron? *Journal of Advanced Nursing*, 65 (3): 663–71.

Bradshaw, A and Price, L (2007) Rectal suppository insertion: the reliability of the evidence as a basis for nursing. *Practice Journal of Clinical Nursing*, 16: 98–103.

Burgoon, JD, Buller, DB and Woodall, W G (1996) *Non-verbal communication: the unspoken dialogue* (2nd edn). New York: Harper Row.

Carr, W and Kemmis, S (1986) *Becoming critical: education, knowledge and action research*. Lewes: Falmer.

Chiseri-Strater, E and Stone Sunstein, B (2006) *Field working: reading and writing research* (3rd edn). Upper Saddle River NJ: Blair Press.

Churpek, MM, Yuen, TC, Huber, MT, Park, SY, Hall, JB and Edelson, DP (2012) Predicting cardiac arrest on the wards: a nested case-control study. Chest, 141 (5): 1170–6.

Coffey, A and Atkinson, P (1996) *Making sense of qualitative data*. London: Sage.

Coulthard, MG, Long, DA, Ullman, AJ and Ware, RS (2012) A randomised controlled trial of Hartmann's solution versus half normal saline in postoperative paediatric instrumentation and craniotomy patients. *Archives of Disease in Childhood*, 97 (6): 491–6.

Creswell, J (2007) *Qualitative inquiry and research design: choosing among five approaches* (2nd edn). Thousand Oaks CA: Sage.

Crotty, M (1998) *The foundations of social research: meaning and perspective in the research process*. London: Sage.

Dearnley, C (2005) A reflection on the use of semi-structured interviews. *Nurse Researcher*, 13 (1): 19–28.

Djivre, SE, Levin, E, Schinke, RJ and Porter, E (2012) Five residents speak: the meaning of living with dying in a long-term care home. *Death Studies*, 36 (6): 487–518.

Doyle, B, Fitzsimons, D, McKeown, P and McAloon, T (2012) Understanding dietary decision-making in patients attending a secondary prevention clinic following myocardial infarction. *Journal of Clinical Nursing*, 21 (1): 32–41.

Dreyfus, H (1991) *Being-in-the-world: a commentary on Heidegger's Being and Time, Division I*. Cambridge MA: The MIT Press.

Ellis, P (2013) *Evidence-based nursing practice* (2nd edn). London: Sage/Learning Matters.

Ellis, PA and Cairns, HS (2001) Renal impairment in elderly patients with hypertension and diabetes. *Quarterly Journal of Medicine*, 94: 261–5.

Fry, M (2012) An ethnography: understanding emergency nursing practice belief systems. *International Emergency Nursing*, 20 (3): 120–5.

Glaser, B and Strauss, A (1967) *The Discovery of Grounded Theory*. Chicago IL: Aldine.

Gomm, R (2000a) Would it work here? in Gomm, R and Davies, C (eds) *Using evidence in health and social care*. London: Sage.

Gomm, R (2000b) Should we afford it?, in Gomm, R and Davies, C (eds) *Using evidence in health and social care*. London: Sage.

Gordis, L (2008) *Epidemiology* (4th edn). Philadelphia PA: Saunders.

Hek, G and Moule, P (2011) *Making sense of research: an introduction for health and social care practitioners* (4th ed.). London: Sage.

Henderson, DK (1993) *Interpretation and explanation in the human sciences*. New York: State University of New York Press.

Hennekens, CH and Buring, JE (1987) *Epidemiology in medicine*. Boston MA: Little Brown and Company.

Henwood, KL and Pidgeon, NR (1992) Qualitative research and psychological theorising. *British Journal of Psychology*, 83 (1): 97–112.

Hinder, S and Greenhalgh, T (2012) This does my head in. Ethnographic study of self management by people with diabetes. *BMC Health Services Research*, 12 (1): 83.

Hobbs, JA (2012) Newly qualified midwives' transition to qualified status and role: assimilating the 'habitus' or reshaping it? *Midwifery*, 28 (3): 391–9.

Hoe, NY and Nambiar, R (1985) Is preoperative shaving really necessary? *Annals of Academic Medicine Singapore*, 14: 700–4.

Holbrook, K (2007) A triangulation study of the clinician and patient experiences of the use of the immunosuppressant drugs azathioprine and 6-mercaptopurine for the management of inflammatory bowel disease. *Journal of Clinical Nursing*, 16 (8): 1427–34.

Horne, G, Seymour, J and Paine, S (2012) Maintaining integrity in the face of death: a grounded theory to explain the perspectives of people affected by lung cancer about the expression of wishes for end of life care. *International Journal of Nursing Studies*, 49 (6): 718–6.

Isoyama, D, Barchi Cordts, E, de Souza van Niewegen, AMB, de Almeida Pereira de Carvalho, W and Parente Barbosa, C (2012) Effect of acupuncture on symptoms of anxiety in women undergoing in vitro fertilisation: a prospective randomised controlled study. *Acupuncture in Medicine*, 3 (2): 85–8.

Koruth, N, Nevison, C and Schwannuer, M (2012) A grounded theory exploration of the onset of anorexia in adolescence. *European Eating Disorders Review*, 20 (4): 257–64.

Kreinin, A, Novitski, D, Rabinowitz, D, Weizman, A and Grinshpoon, A (2012) Associations between tobacco smoking and bipolar affective disorder: clinical, epidemiological, cross-sectional, retrospective study in outpatients. *Comprehensive Psychiatry*, 53 (3): 269–74.

Last, JM (1995) *A dictionary of epidemiology* (3rd edn). Oxford: Oxford University Press.

Lewin, K (1946) Action research and minority problems, in Lewin, GW (ed.) *Researching social conflicts, selected papers on group dynamics*. New York: Harpers.

Lorentzen, V, Dyeremose, V and Larsen, BH (2012) Severely overweight children and dietary changes – a family perspective. *Journal of Advanced Nursing*, 68 (4): 878–87.

Lukkarinen, H (2005) Methodological triangulation showed the poorest quality of life in the youngest people following treatment of coronary artery disease: a longitudinal study. *International Journal of Nursing Studies*, 42: 619–27.

Machin, AI, Machin, T and Pearson, P (2012) Maintaining equilibrium in professional role identity: a grounded theory study of health visitors' perceptions of their changing professional practice context. *Journal of Advanced Nursing*, 68 (7): 1526–37.

Macnee, CL and McCabe, S (2008) *Understanding nursing research: reading and using research in evidence based practice* (2nd edn). London: Wolters Kluwer/Lippincott Williams & Wilkins.

Macneill, V (2009) Forming partnerships with parents from a community development perspective: lessons learnt from Sure Start. *Health and Social Care in the Community*, 17 (6): 659–65.

Martinez-Ramirez, MJ, Delgado-Martinez, AD, Ruiz-Bailen, M, de la Feunte, C, Martinez-Gonzalez, MA and Delgado-Rodriguez, M (2012) Protein intake and fracture risk in elderly people: a case-control study. *Clinical Nutrition*, 31 (3): 391–5.

McNeil, R, Guirguis-Younger, M, Dilley, LB, Aubry, TD, Turnbull, J and Hwang, SW (2012) Harm Reduction Services as a point-of-entry to and source of end-of-life care and support for homeless and marginally housed persons who use alcohol and/or illicit drugs: a qualitative analysis. *BMC Public Health*, 12: 312.

Meeuwsen, EJ, Melis, RJ, Van Der Aa, GC, Goulke-Willemse, GA et al. (2012) Effectiveness of dementia follow-up care by memory clinics or general practitioners: randomised controlled trial. *British Medical Journal*, 344: e3086.

Meffe, F, Moravac, CC and Espin, S (2012) An interprofessional education pilot program in maternity care: findings from an exploratory case study of undergraduate students. *Journal of Interprofessional Care*, 26 (3): 183–8.

Moran, D (2000) *Introduction to phenomenology*. Oxford: Routledge.

Nakstad, AR, Skaga, NO, Pillgram-Larsen, J, Gran, B and Heier, HE (2011) Trends in transfusion of trauma victims: evaluation of changes in clinical practice. *Scandinavian Journal of Trauma, Resuscitation and Emergency Medicine*, 19 (1): 23–31.

Nicholson, WJ, Perkel, G and Selikoff, IJ (1982) Occupational exposure to asbestos: population at risk and projected mortality-1980–2030. *American Journal of Industrial Medicine*, 982 (3): 259.

Nomura, M, Makimoto, K, Kato, M, Shiba, T, Matsuura, C, Shigenobu, K, et al. (2009) Empowering older people with early dementia and family caregivers: a participatory action research study. *International Journal of Nursing Studies*, 46: 431–41.

NRES (National Research Ethics Service) (2008) *NRES information paper on informed consent in clinical trials of investigational medicinal products* (version 3). Available online at: www.nres.npsa.nhs.uk/applications/guidance/consent-guidance-and-forms/?1311929_entryid62=67013 (accessed 2 July 2012).

Nursing and Midwifery Council (NMC) (2008) *The Code: Standards of conduct, performance and ethics for nurses and midwives*. London: NMC.

Nursing and Midwifery Council (NMC) (2010) *Standards for Pre-registration Nursing and Education*. London: NMC.

Parahoo, K (2006) *Nursing research: principles, process and issues* (2nd edn). London: Palgrave Macmillan.

Patrick, J (1973) *A Glasgow gang observed*. London: Methuen.

Patton, M (1986) *How to use qualitative methods in evaluation*. London: Sage.

Patton, M (2002) *Qualitative research and evaluation methods* (3rd edn). London: Sage.

Pesonen, AK, Raikkonen, K, Heinonen, K, Kajantie, E, Forsén, T and Eriksson JG (2007) Depressive symptoms in adults separated from their parents as children: a natural experiment during World War II. *American Journal of Epidemiology*, 166 (10): 1126–33.

Peterson, ER and Barron KA (2007) How to get focus groups talking: new ideas that will stick. *International Journal of Qualitative Methods*, 6 (3):140–4.

Polkinghorne, DE (1989) Phenomenological research methods, in Valle, RS and Halling, S (eds), *Existential-phenomenological perspectives in psychology: exploring the breadth of human experience*. New York: Plenum Press.

Popay, J, Rogers, A and Williams, G (1998) Rationale and standards for the systematic review of qualitative literature in health services research. *Qualitative Health Research*, 8 (3): 341–51.

Powney, J and Watts, M (1987) *Interviewing in educational research*. London: Routledge & Kegan Paul.

Raanaas, RK, Patil, GG and Hartig, T (2012) Health benefits of a view of nature through a window: a quasi-experimental study of patients in a residential rehabilitation center. *Clinical Rehabilitation*, 26 (1): 21–32.

Robson, C (2006) Evaluation research, in Gerish, K and Lacey, A (eds) *The research process in nursing* (5th edn). Oxford: Blackwell.

Rowley, J and Taylor, B (2011) Dying in a rural residential aged care facility: an action research and reflection project to improve end-of-life care to residents with a non-malignant disease. *International Journal of Nursing Practice*, 17: 591–8.

Sackett, DL, Rosenberg, WM, Gray, JA, Haynes, RB and Richardson, WS (1996) Evidence based medicine: what it is and what it isn't. *British Medical Journal*, 312 (7023): 71–2.

Sarantakos, S (2005) *Social Research* (3rd ed). London: Palgrave Macmillan.

Smith, DW (2004) Phenomenology, in Zalta EN (ed) *The Stanford encyclopedia of philosophy* (Summer 2004 edition). Available online at: http://plato.stanford.edu/archives/sum2004/entries/phenomenology/ (accessed 18 December 2009).

Smith, JA and Osborn, M (2004) Interpretative phenomenological analysis, in Smith, JA (ed) *Qualitative psychology*. London: Sage.

Spagrud, LJ, Piira, T and von Baeyer, CL (2003) Children's self-report of pain intensity: the Faces Pain Scale – Revised. *American Journal of Nursing*, 103 (12): 62–4.

Spradley, JP (1980) *Participant observation*. New York: Holt, Rinehart and Wilson.

Starc, G and Strel, J (2012) Influence of the quality implementation of a physical education curriculum on the physical development and physical fitness of children. *BMC Public Health*, 12: 61.

Storesund, A and McMurray, A (2009) Quality of practice in an intensive care unit (ICU): A mini-ethnographic case study. *Intensive and Critical Care Nursing*, 25: 120–7.

Strauss, A and Corbin, J (1990) *Basics of qualitative research*. Thousand Oaks CA: Sage.

Streubert Speziale, HJ and Carpenter, DR (2007) *Qualitative research in nursing: advancing the humanistic imperative* (4th ed.). London: Lippincott Williams & Wilkins.

Tebbet, M and Kennedy, P (2012) The experience of childbirth for women with spinal cord injuries: an interpretative phenomenology analysis study. *Disability and Rehabilitation*, 34 (9): 762–9.

Tedlock, B (2001) Ethnography and ethnographic representation, in Denzin, N and Lincoln, Y (eds) *The handbook of qualitative research*. Thousand Oaks CA: Sage.

Tod, A (2006) Interviewing, in Gerish, K and Lacey, A (eds) *The Research Process in Nursing* (5th edn). Oxford: Blackwell.

Watson, TJ (2012) Narratives in society, organizations and individual identities: an ethnographic study of pubs, identity, work and the pursuit of 'the real'. *Human Relations*, 65 (6): 683–704.

Whiting, LS (2008) Semi-structured interviews: guidance for novice researchers. *Nursing Standard*, 22 (23): 35–40.

World Medical Association (2008) Declaration of Helsinki. Available online at: www.wma.net/en/30 publications/10policies/b3/index.html (accessed 15 December 2009).

Writing Group for the Women's Health Initiative Investigators (2002) Risks and benefits of estrogen plus progestin in healthy postmenopausal women: Principal results from the Women's Health Initiative randomized controlled trial. *Journal of the American Medical Association*, 288 (3): 321–33.

Yin, RK (2008) *Case study research: design and methods* (4th edn). Thousand Oaks CA: Sage Publications.

Zahavi, D (2003) *Husserl's phenomenology.* Stanford CA: Stanford Press.

Index